A Program of Functional Skills for Activities of Daily Living and Communication

Therapeutic Interventions in Alzheimer's Disease

Second Edition

Joan K. Glickstein, PhD
Glickstein Neustadt, Inc.
Pittsburgh, Pennsylvania

AN ASPEN PUBLICATION®
Aspen Publishers, Inc.
Gaithersburg, Maryland
1997

Glickstein, Joan K.
Therapeutic interventions in Alzheimer's disease : a program of
functional skills for activities of daily living and communication.
Joan K. Glickstein. — 2nd ed.
        p.   cm.
Includes bibliographical references and index.
ISBN 0-8342-0930-6 (alk. paper)
1. Alzheimer's disease—Patients—Rehabilitation.
2. Handicapped—Functional assessment.
I. Title
[DNLM: 1. Alzheimer's Disease—rehabilitation.   2. Activities of Daily Living.
3. Communicative Disorders—in old age.   4. Speech Therapy—methods.
5. Language Therapy—methods.
WT 155 G559t   1997]
RC523.G58   1997
618.97′683—dc21
DNLM/DLC
for Library of Congress   96-45156
CIP

Aspen Publishers, Inc. grants permission for photocopying for limited personal or internal use.
This consent does not extend to other kinds of copying, such as coping for general distribution,
for advertising or promotional purposes, for creating new collective works, or for resale.
For information, address Aspen Publishers, Inc., Permissions Department,
200 Orchard Ridge Drive, Suite 200, Gaithersburg, Maryland 20878.

Orders: (800) 638-8437
Customer Service: (800) 234-1660

About Aspen Publishers • For more than 35 years, Aspen has been a leading professional publisher in a variety of disciplines. Aspen's vast information resources are available in both print and electronic formats. We are committed to providing the highest information available in the most appropriate format for our customers. Visit Aspen's Internet site for more information resources, directories, articles, and a searchable version of Aspen's full catalog, including the most recent publications:
http://www.aspenpub.com
    Aspen Publishers, Inc. • The hallmark of quality in publishing
Member of the worldwide Wolters Kluwer group.

Editorial Resources: Lenda Hill
Library of Congress Catalog Card Number:
ISBN: 0-8342-0930-6

Printed in the United States of America
1   2   3   4   5

Table of Contents

Preface

In the years following the first publication of this book much has changed and much has remained the same. Our knowledge base regarding Alzheimer's disease has exploded. Scientists have confirmed and identified a genetic component in at least one type of the disease, and may be able to determine the presence of the disease through a blood test. Unfortunately, at this time there remains no cure and the course of the disease remains somewhat unpredictable.

Although literally hundreds of books and articles have been written describing management techniques for families, as well as palliative programs for day care centers, assisted living facilities, and nursing homes, there remains a noticeable lack of material directed toward rehabilitation specialists regarding the development of, and reimbursement for, rehabilitation programs for persons with dementia. This book is an exception to that rule.

Since the course of the disease can last more than 15 to 20 years, the better the caregiver and client understand the problem, the better they can work with each other, and the easier the burden for all involved in the treatment and care of the person with dementia. On a more positive note, it is now recognized that despite the fact that one cannot reverse or stay ahead of the changes associated with dementia that are taking place in the brain, it does not mean that the dementia client is incapable of learning new behaviors that could improve function in activities of daily living (ADLs) and ultimately the quality of life, or that caregivers cannot learn appropriate rehabilitation/restorative techniques.

To achieve successful outcomes, therapists must know their clients. Because the symptoms and needs of Alzheimer's clients differ, the therapist must first identify those behaviors that can be improved, stabilized, and managed. Formal therapy consumes only a small part of the client's time. Most of the client's time will be spent with a caregiver. For the client in the community, the caregiver is usually a spouse or other family member. However, once the client leaves the home and enters the care of professionals—be it at a nursing facility, assisted living facility, or day care center—care is generally provided by an aide or volunteer under the supervision of a professional. Regardless of the setting, it is imperative that caregivers understand that, although there is no magic bullet, setting up a system of management for ADLs and communication can help to ease the burden for everyone. Therefore, effective therapy for the Alzheimer's client must include the caregiver.

Many family members are creative and develop helping strategies as the need arises. Based on experience with families, clients, laypersons, and professionals, this book has been written to help professionals develop an action plan. The strategies presented here, all of which have been reported by caregivers and therapists, are systematized so that a professional can teach both caregiver and client how to maintain ADLs and communication at the highest functional level throughout the course of the disease.

As the disease progresses, it becomes more and more difficult for the Alzheimer's client to handle day-to-day tasks and to learn new strategies. By analyzing the functional needs—dressing, shopping, and so forth—of Alzheimer's clients living in the community, I have developed a set of alternative strategies that the individual client and caregiver can practice before they are needed rather than waiting until a particular skill is lost. The lessons in Unit 8 are designed to be used by a professional working with Alzheimer's clients who are able to follow simple basic commands, as well as by the caregivers or individuals who are directly responsible for the clients' well-being. None of the lessons requires more than 50 minutes in the therapy situation. Outside of the therapy situation, practice involves the use of a learned strategy during an actual event, which may require only 5 or 10 minutes. Obviously, if the caregiver and client do not go shopping, they will not need to undertake the lesson dealing with the skills related to that task. On the other hand, all clients need strategies to manage daily routines. Therefore, practice takes place not in a contrived situation, but when the client is actually performing a task.

In addition to the lessons described above, a new program has been added: the Action Oriented Program for Persons with Cognitive Disabilities (AOPPCD). This program was developed for long-term care residents who are in the middle to late stages of the disease. Using the Glickstein Neustadt Functional Maintenance Therapy system, the reader learns how to develop reimbursable Functional Maintenance Programs. The chapter on reimbursement has been expanded to include the federal regulations approving therapy for persons with Alzheimer's disease.

Occupational therapists working to improve their clients' ADLs can use the lessons as presented, with minimal adaptation to the environment. Home care professionals will find that the lessons simplify complex tasks by offering a step-by-step approach. Ultimately, of course, the client and the caregiver need the kind of skills outlined in the lessons. Including the caregiver as an adjunct therapist or partner in the lesson guarantees the follow up needed for success.

Happily, when presenting these materials it is no longer necessary to ask, is this relevant to language and communication? In 1907, when Alois Alzheimer first described the disease that now bears his name, aphasia was included among the symptoms present in these patients. Cummings, Benson, Hill, and Read (1985), in a study of aphasia in dementia of the Alzheimer's type, found language abnormalities in all of the Alzheimer's subjects, and a consistent relationship between increased impairment of language function and increased severity of dementia. Others have come to similar conclusions.

Is this traditional speech/language therapy? Absolutely not. It is functional communication therapy, which is what speech/language therapy is all about. The essence of this approach is to reduce the end product of communication to a specific functional outcome, such as eating or shaving or using the telephone. Although some traditional speech/language therapy methods such as matching words and objects are used for higher level clients, the functional communication therapy lessons require the presence of a third party, revolve around the client's daily activities, and are based on functional outcomes.

Alzheimer's disease is no longer a neglected or "orphan" disease. Increasingly, therapists from various disciplines are working with this population. The sudden rush to provide service where none existed before has created both a need and an opportunity for all health care professionals working with Alzheimer's clients. The need is for trained personnel and training materials that go beyond the palliative; the opportunity is to create truly interdisciplinary teams that will make the continuum of care a reality.

Acknowledgment

Any book intended to be understood and used by others would be impossible to complete without help; this book is no exception. In recognition of the many hours spent editing, consulting, reviewing, and mothering, I would like to say a special thank you to my friend and colleague Shirley Schultz.

I would also like to thank the staff of Glickstein Neustadt, Inc. (GNI) who helped to develop and test the AOPPCD; Lisa Arnold, OTR, and Kathleen Kovka, SLP, CCC, who spent many additional hours developing forms, offering suggestions, and overseeing the program; and Alicia Graham, COTA, and Nada Puskaric, SLP, CCC, for their insights and suggestions and for making the program work.

As a final note, I would like to thank my partner, Gail Neustadt, who identified the theory and helped me put it all in perspective.

Introduction

This book is directed toward professionals working with dementia clients, particularly those professionals who are working one-on-one with dementia clients and their caregivers. The overall goal is to provide health care professionals with therapy material that can be used in the development of individualized programs suitable for use with this client population. To facilitate this goal, the text has been divided in three main parts.

Part I is a general overview of aging and Alzheimer's disease. This section provides the reader with a working familiarity with current terminology, diagnostic determination and work-ups, management strategies, and theories of disease causation and progression. Information related to family needs is also provided.

Part II, developed in response to the needs of professionals seeking therapy techniques suitable for dementia clients, is a workbook consisting of a series of specific lesson plans that can be adjusted to the client's changing functional level, and repeated as appropriate. This approach to therapy is unique in that the caregiver is used as an adjunct therapist to ensure the follow up of the lessons and to improve, by practice, the client's interactive communication skills. Another distinguishing feature of this approach to therapy is the definition of caregiver. In all of the lessons, the caregiver is defined as any significant other having close contact with the individual with dementia who is willing to accept the role. No prior training or specific skills are needed. The caregiver for the dementia client living at home is frequently a spouse, but may be someone else living in the home. For the client who is institutionalized, an aide or nurse having frequent contact with the individual may be designated as the caregiver. The therapist trains both the client and the caregiver during the lesson. Language considerations and instruments used to measure functional skills are also discussed in Part II. Finally, the reader will find information regarding methods of documenting the lessons, as well as a general discussion of current reimbursement mechanisms.

Part III offers some practical suggestions that the health care professional will find useful. Those wishing to prepare their own therapy materials to use with dementia clients can turn to Appendix C for a "how-to" description.

The rationale for the development of the workbook presented in Part II is supported by a number of studies. Kirshner, Webb, Kelly, and Wells (1984) found that, although the most prominent initial symptom of Alzheimer's disease is memory disorder, the first manifestation of the disease may be a language disorder. On the other hand, Crystal, Horoupian, Katzman, and Jotkowitz (1982) and Nissen, Corkin, Buonanno, Growdon, Wray, and Bauer (1985) found that a visual spatial disorder or another behavioral disorder, such as a change in personality, may present as the initial problem. Despite variations in the order of appearance and the pattern of predominance among cognitive deficits as the disease progresses, all clients develop a disorder of naming that remains a prominent factor in determining communication strategies (Sjogren, 1952; Appell, Kertesz, & Fisman, 1982; Cummings et al., 1985).

In a study involving repeated testing of a group of ten clients with Alzheimer's disease, Corkin, Growdon, Sullivan, and Shedlack (1981) found that even clients with dementia could derive lasting benefits from practice. On the basis of this evidence, these investigators concluded that clients with mild to moderate Alzheimer's disease can acquire new information and retain it. They postulated that "This benefit from experience in the laboratory setting can be extrapolated to the expectation that appropriate regimens might improve cognitive function or competence in activities for daily living" (Corkin et al., 1981, p. 246).

In 1986, McEvoy and Patterson compared the progress of a group of elderly patients with dementia at a short-term residential treatment facility with a group of elderly psychiatric patients who were not demented. Both groups were treated in a behavioral program designed to retrain them in skills needed for noninstitutional living. The investigators found that demented subjects' improvement was comparable to that of the nondemented subjects in several areas, including communication and some ADL skills. They concluded that their study ". . . does suggest that a diagnosis of dementia should not preclude the possibility that some skills that appear to be lost can be acquired again by certain patients" (pp. 477–478).

The lesson plans presented in this book are based on the above findings and on my own extensive experience working with Alzheimer's clients and their families. Over the years, I have identified a number of verbal and nonverbal behaviors that are here refined into a series of basic lessons aimed at establishing and maintaining functional skills necessary for daily activities. All extraneous stimuli have been eliminated from the lessons to allow the client maximum opportunity for success. Each task is outcome oriented. The goal of each lesson is to improve or maintain function.

The lesson plans take advantage of the client's current abilities in order to prepare him or her for the losses that will occur at the disease progresses. By training both the client and the caregiver to use alternative strategies before they are needed, neither will have to learn a new strategy when the old one is no longer feasible.

In an effort to locate therapy materials suitable for the dementia client, I found that, although books and pamphlets offering information and advice regarding the nature of Alzheimer's disease have proliferated, there are no systematic lesson plans or standardized materials available to the professional working with the dementia client. Part II is designed to fill the gap.

Hopeless and helpless are two words frequently used by professionals when describing Alzheimer's survivors. In my close association with many Alzheimer's survivors and their families I have learned that we expect the worst, hope for the best, and help one another as best as we can.

Part I

EVALUATION AND MANAGEMENT OF DEMENTIA CLIENTS

Overview of Aging and Dementia

DEMOGRAPHICS AND CURRENT TRENDS IN AGING

There are many ways to define "aging." There is physiological aging of an organism, which, some argue, begins as soon as the organism comes into being. There is also behavioral and sociological aging, which involves changes apart from those that may be purely physical. The most common association with the term aging, however, is changes that occur with the passage of time. It is this type of aging, chronological aging, that will be referred to here in the discussion of demographics and current trends. In keeping with the terms used by the U.S. government with regard to the "older population," those 55–64 years of age are designated as "approaching older ages," those 65–74 years of age are "young old," those 75–84 years of age are "old," and those 85 and older are "oldest-old" (U.S. Department of Health and Human Services, April, 1995).

The proportion of the population comprising older persons has grown from less than 10% at the beginning of this century to 20% in 1982. This growth is expected to continue into the next century. According to the U.S. Bureau of the Census (1982), by the year 2050 one of every three persons will be more than 55 years of age, and one of every four persons will be more than 65 years of age. These projections are based on three assumptions: (1) fertility rates will remain steady, (2) life expectancy will rise slowly, and (3) net immigration into the United States will remain at 450,000 persons per year. An increase in any of the three basic assumptions on which these statistics are based will cause the projections to be understated.

Contrary to popular belief, the primary cause of the "graying of America" is not increased longevity; the rise in the absolute number of elderly persons is attributable to the "baby booms" before 1920 and after World War II (U.S. Senate Special Committee on Aging, 1983). Increased longevity is considered a secondary or contributing cause.

In the last 20 years, efforts to assess the health status of the older population have shifted from measuring mortality rates to measuring functional disability. According to Brody and Ruff (1986), chronic illness that results in functional disability is the major health problem of today's elderly. Chronic conditions are relatively rare in younger age groups, but account for the majority of disabilities by middle age. The leading chronic conditions for the older population in 1989 were arthritis, hypertension, hearing impairments, and heart disease (U.S. Senate Special Committee on Aging, 1991).

Although most older persons are able to live independently, severe effects of chronic illness do prevent many individuals from achieving independence, which in turn increases the need for long-term care services. The rate of nursing home use by the elderly has almost doubled since the introduction of Medicare and Medicaid in 1966, from 2.5% to 5% of the population over age 65. It is likely that this number will continue to increase primarily because of the growth in the proportion of people over age 85. Current projections indicate that from 1990 to the year 2005, the nursing home population will increase from 1.5 million to 2.1 million, and further increase to 2.6 million by 2020 (U.S. Senate Special Committee on Aging, 1991).

Impairment in function, which limits independence, is also a risk factor in mortality. According to data from the Longitudinal Study of Aging (LSOA), the risk of death varies with age and degree of functional limitation in ADLs or instrumental activities of daily living (IADLs) (U.S. Department of Health and Human Services, 1995, p. 6). For persons 70–79 years of age with no limitation in ADLs in 1984, 20% were known to have died by 1990, regardless of their IADL limitation. The risk of death was 2.5 times greater for those with a limitation in at least one ADL and 3 times greater for those persons with three or more ADL limitations. Limitations in three or more ADLs are of interest because they are often seen as a trigger for long-term care.

The risk of death was also associated with IADL limitations, regardless of ADL limitation. There was a twofold increase in risk for death with limitation in one or more IADLs for persons 70–79 years of age and a threefold increase if there were three or more IADLs affected. For persons who were alive at the time of the LSOA recontact in 1990, having any limitation in ADL increased the risk of having a hospital stay, a nursing home stay, or both by the 1990 recontact. Seventy-five percent of persons alive in 1990 who had ADL difficulty in 1984 had a hospital or nursing home stay during the interim period, compared with only 55% of those with no ADL difficulties in 1984. The crisis in long-term care has become an issue of national concern, and those in the health care professions must be prepared to meet the present challenges as well as those that lie ahead.

MISCONCEPTIONS AND REALITIES ABOUT AGING

The general public holds a number of misconceptions about aging and mental abilities in America. This becomes obvious when the terms "senility," "dementia," and "Alzheimer's disease" are used interchangeably. Health care professionals must be aware that it is the misconceptions that frequently act as barriers to effective care for the old and for those diagnosed as having Alzheimer's disease.

Senility

One erroneously held idea is that, if one lives long enough, senility cannot be avoided. This idea is partially based on fact and partially on ignorance and a stereotyped image of old people. Senility, or a marked loss of cognitive abilities, was once considered a normal part of the aging process. Scientists have now shown that senility, more accurately termed dementia, is not a normal part of aging. The first case of Alzheimer's disease, which is one type of dementia, was identified in a 51-year-old woman. Dementia afflicts about 5% of individuals over the age of 65, 20% of those at age 80, and 30% of those at age 90. The converse is that 70% of people at age 90 are cognitively normal (Rabins, 1984).

Health Problems

Old people are believed to get sick more often than young people. Although it is true that the incidence of chronic illness increases with age, the incidence of acute conditions decreases. Most older Americans assess their health favorably, even though they may have a physical limitation (U.S. Senate Special Committee on Aging, 1991). As the aging population increases, there is bound to be a large number of individuals in need of health-related and other services, but numbers alone can offer a distorted view of reality.

Misconceptions persist regarding the health problems of the older population and whether those problems become more serious with increasing age. According to the results of the 1989 Health Interview Survey conducted by the National Center for Health Statistics, nearly 71% of elderly people living in the community described their health as excellent, very good, or good, compared with others their age; only 29% reported fair or poor health (U.S. Senate Special Committee on Aging, 1991, p. 108). In an earlier survey conducted by the National Council on Aging (NCOA), 3,427 Americans of all ages were asked to categorize ten problems according to whether they considered them "very serious," "somewhat serious," or "hardly a problem at all," first for themselves and again for persons over the age of 65. Younger respondents perceived all ten problems as far more serious for the elderly than did the elderly respondents themselves (U.S. Senate Special Committee on Aging, 1984).

The commonly held notion that older people's problems are different from those of younger people was also found to be without basis by the NCOA study. With few exceptions, the responses of older and younger persons were similar when rating ten problems in order of importance to themselves. All ages ranked "fear of crime," "not having enough money to live on," and "poor health" as the most serious problems for them personally. The exceptions occurred in the following areas. "Not enough job opportunities" was seen as a serious problem by more young persons than older individuals. "Poor health" and "loneliness" were considered serious problems by more persons over the age of 65 than by persons between the ages of 18 and 65.

Isolation

Although older people report "loneliness" to be among their serious problems, they are not alone and isolated. Approximately 30% of all persons 65 years and older live alone. Contrary to the idea that most older persons do not have contact with their children, data from a national survey demonstrated that most older people lived relatively close to at least one of their children and had frequent contact with them. Only 11% of those surveyed had not seen a child in the previous month. Neighbors and relatives other than children also provide support.

As a group, older people are more likely to vote, and they volunteer their time and abilities more frequently than younger persons. In 1981 the National Center for Education Statistics (NCES) found that 2.5 million persons over 55 years of age participated in adult education courses. Contrary to popular belief, withdrawal from society and a lack of interest in outside activities are not a normal part of the aging process. Americans are just beginning to realize that senior citizens represent a vast resource, not a liability.

Nursing Homes

Another misconception is that, because of the physiological deterioration caused by aging, we can all expect to wind up in nursing homes. There is a certain degree of resentment implicit in this belief that may be attributable to the high cost we all must pay in terms of increased taxes and reduced services to the young in order to maintain individuals beyond a certain age. Other implications are that "old" means useless, dependent, and helpless.

Of course, there are many changes associated with aging. Physiologically, there are decreases in bone mass, muscle strength, vision, hearing, sense of smell, and ability to judge pain. There is an increase in chronic ailments such as arthritis. Although most older persons have at least one chronic condition, only 5% of the population age 65 or older is in a nursing home on a given day. In terms of selective age groups residing in nursing homes, 1% of persons 65 to 74 years of age and 22% of persons 85 or older are in nursing homes. Thus, almost 80% of individuals over 85 years of age are at home.

When the elderly were asked to compare their health with others of their own age, only 8% described their health as comparably poor. Ninety-two percent described their health as good or excellent compared to others (Harris, 1981). Economically, however, older adults do have the highest per capita health expenses of any segment of the population (Health Care Finance Administration, 1982).

Psychiatric Disorders

The mental health problems of older persons are significant in their potential influence on the course of physical illness. It is generally believed that older people with psychiatric disorders do not benefit from therapies as much as younger people. Estimates of the incidence of mental health or psychiatric problems among the elderly generally range from 15% to 25% for persons 65 years and older, which is approximately the same as that for the general public. The number of people with mental disorders living in nursing homes continues to rise. At the same time, 27% of state mental hospital patients are age 65 or older. (U.S. Senate Special Committee on Aging, 1991).

The primary mental health problem of older people was found to be cognitive impairment. Cognitive impairment, whether from Alzheimer's disease or other causes, is one of the principal reasons for institutionalization. The rate for mild impairment, however, was substantially higher (14% for both males and females) than for severe impairment (5.6% for males and 3% for females). Failure in cognitive function is one of the principal reasons for institutionalization of the elderly, with 22% of nursing home residents having a primary diagnosis of a mental disorder or senility without psychosis (U.S. Senate Special Committee on Aging, 1984). On the basis of these statistics, 25% of all elderly Americans have some degree of cognitive impairment. On the other hand, 75% of all elderly Americans have no cognitive impairment.

Summary

Aging is a complex and natural process, not an illness or disease. Although it is true that the longer one lives the closer one is to death, a look at chronological aging alone offers little insight into the actual needs and potential of an individual. Understanding the aging process requires that it be viewed on a multidimensional continuum that includes sociological, physiological, psychological, and chronological changes. Each individual has unique and different needs at different points on the continuum.

Contrary to common beliefs, the majority of America's older population remains independent, alert, and relatively healthy despite limitations and chronic illness. With few exceptions, the needs of the older population are the same as those of the younger population. Unfortunately, for those in need of health care, accessing and surviving a health care system filled with misconceptions can be a heroic odyssey.

DEMENTIA AND ALZHEIMER'S DISEASE

Overview of Dementia

Although in the discussion above the terms "senility," "dementia," and "Alzheimer's disease" were used interchangeably, these terms have specific meanings. The term "senile" literally means "old." In the literal sense, we all grow senile. Over the years, however, the connotation of the word "senile" when applied to an older individual became "out of one's mind" or "demented."

The term "senile dementia" made its first appearance in the nineteenth century and was attributed to dementia that occurred as part of the aging process. In 1898, the term "presenile dementia" was introduced by Binswanger to distinguish younger patients from older ones showing similar progressions of mental deterioration (Lipowski, 1981). Until the twentieth century, references to dementia generally did not distinguish between "organic" and "functional" disorders.

An operational definition of dementia as "an acquired persistent compromise in intellectual function with impairments in at least three of the following spheres of mental activity: language, memory, visuo-spatial skills, personality, and cognition (e.g., abstraction, judgment, mathematics)" allows for differentiation of dementia from other types of intellectual and psychological disturbances, such as mental retardation and depression (Cummings, 1984a). The hallmarks of dementia are memory loss, acquired intellectual deficit, and persistence. The presence of dementia implies an organic disease that is not part of the normal aging process. In some instances dementia is reversible. The current criteria for the diagnosis of dementia of the Alzheimer's type are given in Exhibit 1–1.

Overview of Alzheimer's Disease

Alzheimer's disease is one of many forms of dementia. It accounts for approximately 54% of all cases of dementia. Although a dementia is not always Alzheimer's disease, Alzheimer's disease is always a dementia.

In 1907, the German physician Alois Alzheimer described, in a 51-year-old patient designated as having presenile dementia, the characteristic set of clinical and neuropathological findings of the disease that now bears his name. It was not until 1970, when Tomlinson, Blessed, and Roth published the results of their investigations, that the medical and epidemiological aspects of the disease became known.

Alzheimer's disease, sometimes referred to as AD, is a brain disorder characterized by a progressive dementia. It usually occurs in middle or late life, although on rare occasions it has occurred in young adults. Pathological changes found in autopsy specimens of brains from persons diagnosed as having Alzheimer's disease include degeneration of specific nerve cells, presence of neuritic plaques and neurofibrillary tangles, changes in the forebrain cholinergic systems and, in some cases, changes in the noradrenergic and somatostatinergic systems that innervate the cerebral hemispheres and the basal ganglia. The basal ganglia consist of three nuclei—the caudate nucleus, the globus pallidus, and the putamen—plus the amygdala (Brun, 1983). Adjacent to the amygdala is a structure known as the hippocampus. In Alzheimer's disease, plaques are particularly numerous in the cortex and hippocampus of the brain.

The course of the disease is unrelenting. The onset is slow and insidious, but over time all mental and physical capacities are lost. The progression of the disease can be relatively rapid (5 years from diagnosis to death) or slow (more than 15 years). Since there are no physical illnesses that are routinely associated with the disease, the Alzheimer's patient may appear to be in good health for many years. In fact,

Exhibit 1–1 Diagnostic Criteria for Dementia of the Alzheimer's Type

A. Demonstrable evidence of impairment in short- and long-term memory. Impairment in short-term memory (inability to learn new information) may be indicated by inability to remember three objects after five minutes. Long-term memory impairment (inability to remember information that was known in the past) may be indicated by inability to remember past personal information (e.g., what happened yesterday, birthplace, occupation) or facts of common knowledge (e.g., past presidents, well-known dates).

B. At least one of the following:
  1. impairment in abstract thinking, as indicated by inability to find similarities and differences between related words, difficulty in defining words and concepts, and other similar tasks
  2. impaired judgment, as indicated by inability to make reasonable plans to deal with interpersonal, family, and job-related problems and issues
  3. other disturbances of higher cortical function, such as aphasia (disorder of language), apraxia (inability to carry out motor activities despite intact comprehension and motor function), agnosia (failure to recognize or identify objects despite intact sensory function), and "constructional difficulty" (e.g., inability to copy three-dimensional figures, assemble blocks, or arrange sticks in specific designs)
  4. personality change (i.e., alteration or accentuation of premorbid traits)

C. The disturbance in A and B significantly interferes with work or usual social activities or relationships with others.

D. Not occurring exclusively during the course of delirium.

E. One of the following:
  1. there is evidence from the history, physical examination, or laboratory tests of a specific organic factor (or factors) judged to be etiologically related to the disturbance
  2. in the absence of such evidence, an etiologic organic factor can be presumed if the disturbance cannot be accounted for by any nonorganic mental disorder, such as major depression accounting for cognitive impairment.

Criteria for Severity of Dementia

Mild: Although work or social activities are significantly impaired, the capacity for independent living remains, with adequate personal hygiene and relatively intact judgment.

Moderate: Independent living is hazardous, and some degree of supervision is necessary.

Severe: Activities of daily living are so impaired that continual supervision is required (e.g., unable to maintain minimal personal hygiene; largely incoherent or mute).

Source: Reprinted with permission from the *Diagnostic and Statistical Manual of Mental Disorders,* Fourth Edition. © 1994, American Psychiatric Association.

some Alzheimer's patients are physically healthier than their caregivers. This outward appearance of "wellness" frequently makes it more difficult for family and friends of the patient to accept the cognitive and personality changes that occur.

None of the various symptoms exhibited by the individual is unique to Alzheimer's disease. Many other conditions, both physical and psychological, can present with the same symptoms. Two rare disorders, Pick's disease and Creutzfeldt-Jakob disease, are difficult to differentiate from Alzheimer's disease. Individuals with Pick's disease usually show poor judgment and have predominant behavioral problems early in the course of the disease. As the disease progresses, however, it becomes increasingly more difficult to differentiate between it and Alzheimer's disease. In Creutzfeldt-Jakob disease there may be vague physical complaints, dizziness, nervousness, apathy, irritability, and confusion. This is followed by memory impairment and various neurological signs and symptoms.

In Alzheimer's disease problems of memory, particularly short-term memory, are common in the early stage. In general, the early signs of a possible dementing illness are forgetfulness, repetitiousness, losing one's way, and the loss of ability to perform complex tasks on the job. Of these four signs, the appearance of the last usually signals the need for evaluation. A diagnosis of Alzheimer's disease, based on clinical evidence, is always stated as "probable" Alzheimer's since diagnostic confirmation can be made only on autopsy.

As of this writing, there is no specific drug available to the general public that can stop or reverse the progression of these diseases. Medical management is focused on treating behavioral symptoms and managing the individual's general well-being.

Mortality Trends for Alzheimer's Disease

Epidemiological studies indicate that for individuals over the age of 65, the prevalence of Alzheimer's disease approximately doubles every five years, rising from less than 1% among those 60–65 years of age to as much as 40% in people over the age of 85 (Banner, 1992). Trend data from 1979 through 1991, on deaths from Alzheimer's, show an increasing trend. However, the source data for this trend is not as clear. In 1991, 14,112 Alzheimer's deaths were reported in the United States, 13,768 of which were persons 65 years of age and older, making Alzheimer's the eleventh leading cause of death for individuals 65 years and older. The age–specific death rates for persons 85 years and over were about 19 times greater than those for persons between the ages of 65 and 74 years.

It is interesting to note that the age-adjusted death rate for Alzheimer's, which eliminates the effects of the aging of the population, increased significantly each year from 1979 to 1988. However from 1988 to 1991 there was no statistically significant single-year increase. This trend may have occurred due to any one or a combination of factors. It should be recalled that prior to 1979 very little had been said publicly about this disease. Thinking by both lay persons and a majority of the medical profession held that Alzheimer's disease was a normal part of the aging process—another name for senility or chronic organic brain syndrome. It was not until the 1981 White House Conference on Aging that a spotlight was turned on Alzheimer's disease. At that time, Alzheimer's was specifically targeted as a disease worthy of special attention. Public awareness brought with it public funds for research, which, in turn, brought better diagnostic tools.

Hoyert (1993), in comparing the trends and patterns in reporting mortality from Alzheimer's disease, found similar patterns in records that showed an autopsy was done and those records that showed no autopsy. This suggests that the reason for the increase in reporting has nothing to do with autopsy evidence. It is possible that the increasing awareness of the disease along with increasing diagnosis, as well as other unidentified factors, rather than any substantial changes in the risk of dying from Alzheimer's are likely causes for increased reporting of the disease as a cause of death.

Other trends that have been noted: age-adjusted death rates for the disease are greater for men than women, and greater for the white than the black population (U.S. Department of Health and Human Services, January 1996). Here again, one needs to question the source data. Since, in this country, more white persons seek professional diagnoses and outside support for this disease than persons of color, it is possible that this trend is an artifact of the data collecting system. Researchers in other countries evaluating the occurrence of Alzheimer's in different general populations have found no consistent differences. In general, the rates are about the same throughout the world, and do not appear to depend heavily on race or sex.

Banner (1992, p. 31) states that "for dementias of aging, delay is prevention. . . . Even a delay of 5 years would result in eliminating about 50 percent of the disease, whereas a delay of about 12 years would essentially eliminate AD as a major public health problem."

Conceptual Models of Alzheimer's Disease

To date, the only established risk factors for Alzheimer's disease are age, family history, and genetics. However, most scientists do not believe that these are the only risk factors. Research is focused on six different conceptual models of Alzheimer's disease based on symptoms and pathological findings and on the processes that might give rise to them. The objective is to focus on populations with specific characteristics in an effort to uncover modifiable risk factors and to identify factors that may help to protect against the disease.

Genetic Model

There are a number of ways that a genetic disease can manifest itself. It can stem from an abnormal chromosome or from an inborn error of metabolism, in which an abnormality in the genetic material, DNA, impairs the ability of cells to make a particular protein. Scientists have noted that there are some families in which the incidence of Alzheimer's disease is unusually high. In a series of studies conducted on families from Minnesota, Heston demonstrated an increased risk for secondary cases of Alzheimer's disease in first-degree relatives (Heston, 1977; Heston & White, 1978). Within families, close relatives of a person with Alzheimer's disease (parents and siblings) are about twice as likely to develop the disease as more distant relatives, but not necessarily twice as likely as the public at large.

Heston has stressed that estimates of empirical risk, the statistical chance a person has of getting the disease, is age specific. The risks are higher in those families where the disease starts before age 65 than in families where it starts later. Heston and collaborators (Heston & Mastri, 1977; Heston, 1979) also noted increased risk of Down syndrome, lymphoproliferative cancers, autoimmune disorders, and other problems related to immune function in families where there was an early onset of the disease. Studies such as these have led to the identification of three chromosomes that are associated with Alzheimer's disease. They are chromosomes 21, 14, and 19.

Chromosomes are threadlike structures. Found in every cell nucleus, chromosomes carry the inheritance factors (genes). They are composed of DNA and a protein. A human cell normally contains 46 chromosomes, 22 homologous pairs and one pair of sex chromosomes. In 1987 St. George-Hyslop and colleagues located a defective gene for Alzheimer's disease on chromosome 21 in the same region that contains the gene for brain amyloid, a protein that accumulates abnormally in the brains of individuals with Down syndrome (Goldgaber et al., 1987; Tanzi et al., 1987). These breakthrough results supported the theory that at least one form of Alzheimer's disease is inherited and that a similar genetic defect may occur in both Alzheimer's disease and Down syndrome. Ongoing studies have shown that both chromosome 21 and chromosome 14 are at fault only in members of relatively rare families with early onset familial Alzheimer's disease (FAD). Researchers now know that people with particular abnormalities in the sequence of their amyloid precursor protein (APP) gene on chromosome 21 are almost certain to develop Alzheimer's disease by the age of 60. Currently, there is no evidence that these chromosomes are associated with cases that occur after age 65 (Goate et al., 1991; Murell et al., 1991; Chartier-Harlin et al., 1991).

A gene involved in late–onset Alzheimer's disease appears to be the APOE (apolipoprotein E) gene on chromosome 19. As the name implies, it is part lipid and part protein. Its known function is to help guide cholesterol around the body and into cells. There are three versions or alleles of this gene termed

APOE-e2, APOE-e3, and APOE-e4. The e4 version (APOE-e4), normally present in about 14% of the population, is much more common in people with late–onset Alzheimer's disease (40–50%) than it is in people without the disease. This is true for people with or without a history of Alzheimer's disease. However, there are many Alzheimer patients who do not have this gene. Because this gene has also been identified in people over the age of 80 who do not have Alzheimer's disease, APOE-e4 has been called a susceptibility gene. Suseptibility genes differ from disease genes in their expression. Unlike the "disease" gene that dictates certainty in the development of the disease, a suseptibility gene increases the risk but often requires other factors to trigger its action. For example, the gene for Huntington's chorea is located on chromosome 4. Inheriting the gene for Huntington's chorea means that the individual will develop the disease. On the other hand, inheriting APOE-e4 increases the odds of developing the disease, but does not mean it will happen.

According to Haney (1996) the discovery of the gene and the risk factors involved, "people born with two E-3 genes develop Alzheimer's 15 years later, on average, than people with two E-4s. With a combination of one E-3 and one E-2, the typical onset is later still." About 2% to 3% of the U.S. population carry two e-4 genes and develop Alzheimer's at age 70. Presence of the relatively rare APOE-e2 gene suggests something quite different. Research suggests that persons with this gene may have a *reduced* risk for the disease.

Abnormal Protein Model

The three major pathologic signs of Alzheimer's disease are (1) neurofibrillary tangles, (2) amyloid that surrounds and invades cerebral blood vessels, and (3) amyloid plaques that replace degenerating nerve terminals (Wurtman, 1985). Each of these signs reflects an accumulation of proteins not normally found in the brain.

(1) Neurofibrillary tangles. Tau protein is a normal component of nerve cells. In Alzheimer's disease tau protein is processed abnormally and forms tangles in nerve cells. Although some neurofibrillary tangles have been found in the brains of persons who had never developed Alzheimer's disease, they are not normally present in large quantities in the human brain, regardless of age. These bundles of fibrous proteins found in neuronal cell bodies are composed, at least in part, of paired helical filaments (PHF), giving rise to the term "tangles." The AD brain tangles are found in the neurites, the long extensions of neurons through which impulses are transmitted to synapses; the hippocampus; and the cerebral cortex. They are also found in brainstem neurons that release neurotransmitters. A major component of the tangles is a protein that normally binds together the microtubules in axons, the neuronal processes that deliver impulses to synapses (Lee et al., 1991). This same type of tangle has been identified in the brains of boxers who have suffered a condition known as "dementia pugilistica" or "punch-drunk syndrome," leading some scientists to conjucture a relationship between head trauma and the onset of Alzheimer's.

(2) Amyloid. Amyloid is a starch-like glycoprotein that can accumulate in body tissue and impair its function. The particular type of amyloid that collects in the brains of persons with Alzheimer's disease is beta-amyloid, a small fragment of a larger protein known as "amyloid precursor protein" or APP. While the structure of APP is known, its normal function is not (Banner, 1992). APP can form various products in different parts of the body. For example, a major product of APP has been identified as "protease nexin-2," a protein that may be involved in blood coagulation. Amyloid is a minor byproduct of APP metabolism that accumulates slowly with age. In the AD brain the amyloid byproduct of APP appears to collect more rapidly and is concentrated at first in the muscular middle layer of a brain blood vessel and advances outward.

(3) Amyloid plaques. Glenner examined a series of 350 brains of patients diagnosed as having Alzheimer's disease premorbidly and found deposits of amyloid plaques in 92% of the brains studied (Wurtman, 1985). The greatest number of amyloid plaques is usually located in the cerebral cortex, the hippocampus, and the amygdala. The number of plaques tends to correlate closely with the extent of dementia.

In addition to accumulating these abnormal proteins, it is hypothesized that the brains of Alzheimer's patients synthesize below-normal quantities of proteins in general. One explanation may be a deficiency of RNA, the nucleic acid that mediates the translation of DNA to manufacture protein. The deficiency in RNA may be due to an improperly regulated enzyme that breaks down the RNA (Wurtman, 1985). There is still no clear explanation in this theory as to why protein accumulation is triggered.

One of the most exciting findings in Alzheimer's research was made by Selkoe and colleagues (1987). Working with aged mammals, the investigators showed that abnormal amyloid plaques are not unique to the human brain, indicating that aged nonhuman primates may serve as animal models for certain aspects of Alzheimer's disease. Banner (1992, p. 34) stresses the importance of learning precisely how amyloid is formed. He states "... It is fairly clear that some step in the processing of APP to form amyloid is pathogenetic for AD. ... The APP biochemical pathway provides a set of potential targets for therapeutic intervention to prevent the development of AD."

Infectious Agent Model

The concept of slow viral infection was originated by Sigurdsson (1954) from his studies of scrapies, a progressive, fatal neurologic disease in sheep. In 1964, a group of scientists led by Gajdusek observed an abnormal structure made up of twisted filaments in the brains of animals with scrapies and people with Creutzfeldt-Jakob disease and kuru.

Creutzfeldt-Jakob disease is a rare progressive form of human dementia that occurs in all parts of the world. Asher and associates were able to transmit Creutzfeldt-Jakob disease from brain tissue of infected humans to chimpanzees after latency periods of up to 4 years (Schneck, Reisberg, & Ferris, 1982). Kuru is a chronic, progressive neurologic disease found in certain tribes in New Guinea. Gajdusek and Gibbs showed that kuru was due to a slow-virus–induced infection with an incubation period measured in years (Gajdusek & Gibbs, 1964; Gibbs & Gajdusek, 1978).

Although the twisted filaments found by Gajdusek and Gibbs are not the same as those in Alzheimer's disease, they do share some immunological properties with the amyloid fibrils of neurofibrillary tangles. Gajdusek and colleagues proposed that this filamentous structure may be the infectious agent in all three diseases.

Toxin Model

Possible toxic causes of dementia include alcohol abuse, heavy-metal poisoning, and poisoning secondary to breathing or eating various compounds. The association of toxins and dementias is neither new nor exclusive to Alzheimer's disease.

The toxin that has received the greatest amount of attention as a possible causative agent in Alzheimer's disease is aluminum. As early as 1965, Klatzo and associates noted the formation of neurofibrillary tangles in rabbit brains that had been injected with aluminum (Klatzo, Wisniewski, & Streicher, 1965). Crapper and Dalton (1973) injected cats with aluminum and noted changes in the animals' behavior. When Crapper and his associates noted similarly elevated levels of aluminum in the autopsied brains of Alzheimer's victims, they postulated that neurofibrillary tangles may be due in part to aluminum intoxication (Crapper, Krishman, & Dalton, 1973) .

Over the years the topic of aluminum as a major factor in Alzheimer's disease has remained controversial. Investigators looking postmorbidly at aluminum levels in the brains of Alzheimer's patients and comparing them with the brains of matched controls have obtained contradictory results. In one study,

McDermott and others (1979) reported no differential increase in aluminum content in Alzheimer's patients and age-matched controls. In contrast, Trapp and associates (1978) found elevated levels in younger or presenile patients but not in older patients or matched controls, posing the possibility of two separate etiologies.

Alfrey and coworkers (1976) found irreversible dementia and high concentrations of aluminum in brain tissue of patients who had undergone repeated kidney dialysis with aluminum-rich salts. These investigators did not find neurofibrillary tangles, however. The relation between the selective accumulation of aluminum and the formation of neurofibrillary tangles in Alzheimer's disease has yet to be explained satisfactorily. Current thinking holds that if aluminum is involved in Alzheimer's disease, it only accounts for a very small number of cases.

Immunological Model

The incidence of Alzheimer's disease increases significantly with age. Both clinical and experimental data suggest that immunological factors may play an important role in Alzheimer's disease, since deterioration in the immune system and a significant increase in the incidence of autoimmune diseases have been associated with aging (Nandy, 1983).

As we age, there is an increase in brain-specific antibodies in the blood serum. This has been observed in both experimental animals and in humans. In 1978, Nandy reported significantly higher levels of such antibodies in some Alzheimer's patients when compared with age-matched controls. Stam and Op Den Velde (1978) found an increase in the expression of one of two genes that are thought to control serum haptoglobins, which may provide a link between immunological and genetic factors. Finding a link between these factors in early-onset Alzheimer's disease does not explain what role immunological factors play. If the deterioration of the immune system is a significant factor in the development of Alzheimer's disease, why doesn't everyone develop it?

Neurochemical Model

One consistent postmortem finding in the brains of individuals who were diagnosed with Alzheimer's disease is a decrease in the neurotransmitter acetylcholine. In 1976, two teams of investigators reported the first clear biochemical abnormality associated with Alzheimer's disease (Davies & Maloney, 1976; Bowen et al., 1979). The demonstration that a specific neurochemical deficit is consistently present in Alzheimer's disease represented a major advance in our understanding of this disease.

While studying the hippocampus and cerebral cortex of Alzheimer's patients, investigators have consistently found the activity of the enzyme choline acetyltransferase (CAT) to be severely reduced (Perry et al., 1977; White et al., 1977). The loss of CAT activity reflects the loss of cholinergic, or acetylcholine-releasing, nerve terminals in these two regions of the brain. This finding suggests an explanation for the primary symptom of the disease, loss of memory. Since cholinergic terminals in the hippocampus are critically important for memory formation, the reduced levels of CAT activity in the hippocampus suggest that the level of acetylcholine (which cannot be measured at autopsy) must also be reduced.

Decreases in acetylcholine metabolism have been shown to correlate with both neuropathological and cognitive changes in Alzheimer's disease (Perry et al., 1977; Perry et al., 1978). Although nerve cells that make acetylcholine seem to be the earliest and most severely affected cells, many other types of nerve cells also deteriorate. Additional neurotransmitters that are depleted include noradrenaline, serotonin, somatostatin, corticotropin releasing factor, and others. Although these and other neurochemical systems have also been reported to be altered in progressive dementia, non-cholinergic neurotransmitter systems appear to be affected to a lesser extent (Reisberg, 1983). The relationship among the neurochemical systems of the body, Alzheimer's disease, and other dementias is not yet fully understood.

EXPERIMENTAL DRUG TREATMENTS

While a number of multiple-neurotransmitter drugs are being evaluated in Alzheimer's disease patients, none has yet shown consistent benefit. One frequently asked question regarding Alzheimer's disease drugs has been "Why haven't these drugs been as successful for AD as L-dopa is for Parkinson's disease?" The response lies in understanding how brain tissue is affected in both diseases. In Parkinson's, dopamine appears to be the major neurotransmitter that is affected. In addition, the depletion of dopamine occurs primarily in a small, focused region of the brain. Contrast this with Alzheimer's disease where widespread degeneration of nerve cells takes place throughout the cerebral cortex involving a large array of neurotransmitters, and it becomes clear why no single drug can accomplish the job. Nevertheless, researchers have tried in various ways to increase the amount of useable acetylcholine in the brain, in the hope that it would improve patients' memory and other abilities for at least some period of time. At best, this is seen as a temporary measure rather than as a cure for the disease. To date, the most successful strategy to augment acetylcholine has been to inhibit its natural breakdown. So far, these drugs have helped only a minority of the Alzheimer's patients who have tried them.

The only drug currently available to the public is Cognex. Cognex is the brand name for tacrine hydrochloride and is referred to in the literature as THA (Physicians Desk Reference, 1996). THA is a cholinesterase inhibitor. Its action is thought to elevate available acetylcholine concentrations in the cerebral cortex by slowing the degradation of acetylcholine released by still intact cholinergic neurons. If this action is correct, the effectiveness of THA will lessen as the disease process progresses and there are fewer cholinergic neurons available. The most serious side effect of this drug is liver damage; patients must be carefully monitored and screened.

Based on the success of Cognex, drug companies are supporting widespread trials of other drugs that act as acetylcholinesterase inhibitors. E2020 and ENA713 are two drugs that appear to be able to improve performance in tests of learning and memory.

SUMMARY

From the study of basic biological properties of nerve cells, and research into injuries and diseases that cause nerve cell degeneration, scientists have learned several processes through which nerve cells can be damaged. While there may be no single cause for Alzheimer's disease it is possible that one or a combination of mechanisms will prove to be the trigger of a "domino effect" of toxic events that culminates in Alzheimer's disease. These mechanisms include deterioration of the outer membrane of the cell, which is vital to the maintenance of the cell; decline in the cell's metabolism, which would limit the cell's ability to repair itself or to carry out its function; injury from free radicals, by-products of normal cell activity that are not removed; and excitotoxic damage, a chain reaction in which nerve cells are overstimulated to the point of destruction.

Although all the models described above help us to understand the disease process, they do not necessarily provide evidence of a direct, causal relationship. We now know that for some cases of Alzheimer's disease there is a genetic component, but genetics alone cannot account for all cases. We also know that the enzyme acetylcholine is sharply decreased and that other enzyme systems are also affected. Nevertheless, investigators are still uncertain as to the causal mechanism of the disease. The more closely scientists look at Alzheimer's disease, the more apparent it becomes that there are probably multiple causative factors of this disease that sometimes differ in younger and older patients (Katzman et al., 1978) and would account for differences in its course and duration.

In reviewing the theories and changes that occur in Alzheimer's disease, it is important to remember that these changes are not exclusive to this disease (Mortimer, 1980). It is possible that in the end Alzheimer's disease may represent a final common neuropathological pathway for many different disease processes.

Clinical and Behavioral Evaluation Procedures in Alzheimer's Disease

Despite a great increase in what is known about the nature of Alzheimer's disease and in the sophistication of new technology for diagnostic procedures, the diagnosis of Alzheimer's disease before death and autopsy remains a process of elimination. A true picture of Alzheimer's disease emerges only over a period of time—frequently more than two years. For this reason, the initial evaluation should be used for comparison purposes with later evaluations. When this is done, the initial evaluation is called the baseline against which changes are measured. Because of the difficulties in diagnosis, it is worth repeating that, although a dementia is not always Alzheimer's disease, Alzheimer's disease is always a dementia. This section discusses evaluation from two views: clinical evaluation of the disease and evaluation based on behavioral changes observed by family members and health care professionals.

In discussing the evaluation of an Alzheimer's client, many individuals automatically think in terms of measuring "decline" or "loss." Evidence of decline or loss does not tell the entire story, however. Anyone wishing to enter into a helping relationship with an Alzheimer's client must remember that a true evaluation will weigh the client's positives as well as negatives.

CLINICAL EVALUATION OF DEMENTIA PATIENTS

Evaluation procedures for persons suspected of having Alzheimer's disease tend to vary depending on the evaluating facility. Some recommended procedures need to be done in a hospital, whereas others can be done on an outpatient basis. Several factors, including financial resources, have a significant bearing on when, where, and to what extent an evaluation will be performed.

Alzheimer's disease is currently diagnosed by eliminating other possible causative factors of dementia. Because there is no specific test for Alzheimer's disease available to the general public, tests are performed for other diseases that produce dementia and present in a similar manner. A partial list of areas to be investigated would include depression, delirium, hypothyroidism, multi-infarct dementia, and chronic alcohol abuse. It is only after these areas are eliminated as causative factors that a diagnosis of probable Alzheimer's disease can be made. Final determination, however, can be made only by examining the brain tissue on autopsy.

Exhibit 2–1 illustrates the criteria developed by a work group on the diagnosis of Alzheimer's disease established by the National Institute of Neurological and Communicative Disorders and Stroke (NINCDS) and the Alzheimer's Disease and Related Disorders Association (ADRDA). The purpose of

---

Exhibit 2–1 Criteria for the Clinical Diagnosis of Alzheimer's Disease

1. The criteria for the clinical diagnosis of PROBABLE Alzheimer's disease include

   dementia established by clinical examination, documented by the Mini-Mental State Examination, Blessed Dementia Scale, or some similar examination, and confirmed by neuropsychological tests;

   deficits in two or more areas of cognition;

   progressive worsening of memory and other cognitive functions;

   no disturbance of consciousness;

   onset between ages 40 and 90, most often after age 65; and

   absence of systemic disorders or other brain diseases that in and of themselves could account for the progressive deficits in memory and cognition.

2. The diagnosis of PROBABLE Alzheimer's disease is supported by

   progressive deterioration of specific cognitive functions such as language (aphasia), motor skills (apraxia), and perception (agnosia);

   impaired activities of daily living and altered patterns of behavior;

   family history of similar disorders, particularly if confirmed neuropathologically; and

   laboratory results of

   normal lumbar puncture as evaluated by standard techniques,

   normal pattern or nonspecific changes in electroencephalogram (EEG), such as increased slow wave activity, and

   evidence of cerebral atrophy on computed tomography with progression documented by serial observation.

3. Other clinical features consistent with the diagnosis of PROBABLE Alzheimer's disease, after exclusion of causes of dementia other than Alzheimer's disease, include

   plateaus in the course of progression of the illness;

continues

Exhibit 2–1 continued

associated symptoms of depression, insomnia, incontinence, delusions, illusions, hallucinations, catastrophic (verbal, emotional, or physical) outbursts, sexual disorders, and weight loss;

other neurologic abnormalities in some patients, especially with more advanced disease and including motor signs such as increased muscle tone, myoclonus, or gait disorder;

seizures in advanced disease; and

computed tomographic scan normal for age.

4. Features that make the diagnosis of PROBABLE Alzheimer's disease uncertain or unlikely include

sudden, apoplectic onset;

focal neurologic findings such as hemiparesis, sensory loss, visual field deficits, and incoordination early in the course of the illness; and

seizures or gait disturbances at the onset or very early in the course of the illness.

5. Clinical diagnosis of POSSIBLE Alzheimer's disease may be made

on the basis of the dementia syndrome, in the absence of other neurologic, psychiatric, or systemic disorders sufficient to cause dementia, and in the presence of variations in the onset, in the presentations, or in the clinical course;

in the presence of a second systemic or brain disorder sufficient to produce dementia that is not considered to be *the* cause of the dementia, and should be used in research studies when a single, gradually progressive, severe cognitive deficit is identified in the absence of other identifiable cause.

6. Criteria for diagnosis of DEFINITE Alzheimer's disease are

the clinical criteria for PROBABLE Alzheimer's disease and histopathologic evidence obtained from a biopsy or autopsy.

7. Classification of Alzheimer's disease for research purposes should specify features that may differentiate subtypes of the disorder, such as

familial occurrence,

onset before age 65,

presence of trisomy-21, and

coexistence of other relevant conditions, such as Parkinson's disease.

Source: Reprinted from *Neurology,* Vol. 34, pp. 940–944, 1984, by permission of Little, Brown and Company Inc.

the group was to "establish and describe clinical criteria for the diagnosis of Alzheimer's disease of particular importance for research protocols and to describe approaches that would be useful for assessing the natural history of the disease" (McKhann et al., 1984, p. 939). The resulting criteria are compatible with definitions in the Diagnostic and Statistical Manual of Mental Disorders (DSMIII-R) and in the International Classification of Diseases (ICD-9). Although the criteria established by the work group are currently accepted, they must be regarded as subject to change since additional longitudinal studies, confirmed by autopsy, are necessary to establish fully their validity.

Procedures Used in Determining Alzheimer's Disease

Exhibit 2–2 lists the possible components that can serve as a guide or checklist when determining whether or not an individual has been thoroughly evaluated for Alzheimer's disease. Not every individual suspected of having this disease will be given every test item listed. There are many professionals who believe that unless the individual is a candidate for, or is part of, an experimental program there is no need to go beyond a basic evaluation of physical, neurological, and mental status and a computed axial tomography (CT) scan. Regardless of the extent of the evaluation, most clients begin the evaluation process with a visit to a physician who will order the necessary tests. The evaluation will determine whether dementia is present and whether the condition is reversible or irreversible. The physician will then offer a diagnosis based on the findings of the evaluation.

History

Since dementia is the decline of memory and other cognitive functions in comparison with the individual's previous level of function, the client's history is a vital part of the evaluation process. The diag-

---

Exhibit 2–2 Evaluation Checklist for Alzheimer's Disease

— A detailed case history from someone close to the client
— Physical examination
— Evaluation of the client's mental status
— Neurological evaluation
— Laboratory tests (blood chemistry and venereal disease Research Laboratories test)
— Thyroid studies
— Lumbar puncture to evaluate spinal fluid
— Electroencephalogram
— Computed axial tomography (CT) scan
— Positron emission tomographic (PET) scan
— Magnetic resonance imaging (MRI) scan
— Cerebral blood flow
— Neuropsychological assessment of cognitive functioning
— Assessment of functional abilities for self-care and activities of daily living
— Assessment of communication skills

Source: Reprinted with permission from *Neurology,* Vol. 34, pp. 940–944, 1984, by permission of Little, Brown and Company Inc.

nosis of dementia is usually suggested by a history of forgetfulness, repetitiousness, losing one's way in familiar surroundings, and the loss of ability to perform complex tasks on the job. In cases where Alzheimer's disease is suspected, the onset is slow and insidious. People do not go to bed healthy and wake up the next day with symptoms.

In taking the case history the familial history should not be overlooked. The family history should include information regarding relatives that might have had dementia, Down syndrome, lymphomas, autoimmune disorders, and other problems related to immune function. In the case of other family members with dementia, age of onset should be considered.

Physical Examination

A thorough physical examination is an important part of evaluating the individual's current health status. Heart disease, diabetes that may have gone unchecked, and many other physical ailments can be contributing causes in a decline in overall function. Sometimes something as simple as severe constipation, a frequently overlooked condition in many elderly people, has been known to cause behavior changes that are due to chronic pain and discomfort.

Mental Status Examination

Clients in the very early stages of dementia may have normal social conversation and appear to function without difficulty. Because they look and sound well, deficits that occur early in the course of the disease may be missed. The purpose of the mental status examination is to detect the presence of intellectual impairment and to gain some indication as to the degree of the impairment.

A mental status examination should include questions that yield information regarding the individual's orientation to person, place, and time; basic math skills; memory; and attention.

Questions such as "What is your name?" and "Can you tell me where you are now?" are typical of the questions used to determine orientation. In the initial stages it is not common for the individual to be disoriented to person. Early-stage Alzheimer's clients can identify themselves. In advanced stages, however, individuals may become unaware of their own person. It is not unusual to hear a family member report that the Alzheimer's client was noted talking to his or her image in a mirror. Orientation to both time and place tend to be affected earlier than orientation to person. Questions regarding the current month and year are sensitive tests of orientation to time. Kim, Morrow, and Boller (1980), in a study that compared Alzheimer's patients with Huntington's disease patients, found the Alzheimer's patients to be more impaired in their orientation to both time and place than the Huntington's patients.

In our society, one commanding task is control of one's personal finances and checkbook. In Alzheimer's disease, early deterioration in this function together with a lack of awareness is common. Asking clients to do simple subtractions, usually without the benefit of pencil and paper, is one way of assessing simple math skills.

Memory may be assessed by asking the client to remember several objects over a period of time. Persons with dementia do more poorly on memory tasks than matched controls. The memory impairment appears to be global in nature, involving both short- and long-term memory (Sanders & Warrington, 1971; Butters & Cermak, 1980).

Two frequently used quantitative measures of mental status are the Mini-Mental State Examination (Folstein et al., 1975), Exhibit 2–3, and the Short Portable Mental Status Questionnaire (SPMSQ) (Pfeiffer, 1975), Exhibit 2–4. Both tests are designed to be used as initial screening tools to detect the presence of intellectual impairment. Neither test should take more than five or ten minutes to complete. Since factors such as education and ethnic background may influence performance on a mental status test, they must be taken into account when administering and scoring these tests.

Exhibit 2–3 Mini-Mental State Examiniation

	Maximum score	Score	Instructions
Orientation:			
What is the (year) (season) (date) (day) (month)?	5	_____	Ask for the date. Then proceed to ask the other parts of the question. One point for each correct segment of the question.
Where are we: (state) (county) (town) (hospital) (floor)?	5	_____	Ask for the facility then proceed to other parts of the question. One point for each correct segment of the question.
Registration:			
Name three objects (bed, apple, shoe). Ask the patient to repeat them.	3	_____	Name the objects slowly, one second for each. Ask patient to repeat. Score by the number he or she is able to recall. Take time here for him or her to learn the series of objects, up to six trials, to use later for the memory test.
Attention and calculation:			
Count backward by 7s. Start with 100. Stop after five calculations.	5	_____	Score the total number correct (93, 86, 79, 72, 65).
Alternate question:			
Spell the word "world" backward.	5	_____	Score the number of letters in correct order (dlrow = 5, dlorw = 2).
Recall:			
Ask for the three objects used under Registration to be repeated.	3	_____	Score one point for each correct answer, (bed, apple, shoe).
Language:			
1. Naming: Name this object (watch, pencil).	2	_____	Hold the object. Ask patient to name it. Score one point for each correct answer.
2. Repetition: Repeat the following—"No ifs, ands, or buts."	1	_____	Allow one trial only. Score one point for correct answer.
3. Follow a three-stage command: "Take the paper in your right hand, fold it in half, and put it on the floor."	3	_____	Use a blank sheet of paper. Score one point for each part correctly executed.
4. Reading: Read and obey the following: Close your eyes	1	_____	Instruction should be printed on a page. Allow patient to read it. Score by correct response.
5. Writing: Write a sentence.	1	_____	Provide paper and pencil. Allow patient to write any sentence. It must contain a noun and verb and be sensible.
6. Copying: Copy this design. 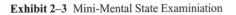	1	_____	All 10 angles must be present. Figures must intersect. Tremor and rotation are ignored.
Total		_____	(Max. 30) Test is not timed.

Source: Reprinted with permission from M.F. Folstein, S.E. Folstein, and P.R. McHugh, Mini-Mental State: A Practical Method for Grading the Cognitive State of Patients for the Clinician, *Journal of Psychological Research,* Vol. 12, pp. 189–198. ©1975, Elsevier Science Ltd. Oxford, England.

Exhibit 2–4 Short Portable Mental Status Questionnaire (SPMSQ)

Instructions: Ask questions 1–10 in this list and record all answers. Ask question 4A only if patient does not have a telephone. Record total number of errors based on 10 questions.

+	−

1. What is the date today? _____
                               Month   Day   Year
2. What day of the week is it? _____
3. What is the name of this place? _____
4. What is your telephone number? _____
4A. What is your street address? _____
   (Ask only if patient does not have a telephone.)
5. How old are you? _____
6. When were you born? _____
7. Who is the president of the United States now? _____
8. Who was president just before him? _____
9. What was your mother's maiden name? _____
10. Subtract 3 from 20 and keep subtracting 3 from each new number, all the way down.

_____ Total Number of Errors

To Be Completed by Interviewer

Patient's Name: _____ Date: _____

Sex: 1. Male   Race: 1. White
     2. Female   2. Black
                         3. Other

Years of Education: _____1. Grade School
                                      2. High School
                                      3. Beyond High School

Interviewer's Name: _____

INSTRUCTIONS FOR COMPLETION OF THE SPMSQ

Ask the subject questions 1 through 10 in this list and record all answers. All responses to be scored as correct must be given by subject without reference to calendar, newspaper, birth certificates, or other aid to memory.

Question 1 is to be scored as correct only when the exact month, exact date, and the exact year are given correctly.

continues

Exhibit 2–4 continued

Question 2 is self-explanatory.

Question 3 should be scored as correct if any description of the location is given. "My home," correct name of the town or city of residence, or the name of hospital or institution if subject is institutionalized, are all acceptable.

Question 4 should be scored as correct when the telephone number can be verified, or when the subject can repeat the same number at another point in the questioning.

Question 5 is scored as correct when stated age corresponds to date of birth.

Question 6 is to be scored as correct only when the month, exact date, and year are all given.

Question 7 requires only the last name of the president.

Question 8 requires only the last name of the previous president.

Question 9 does not need to be verified. It is scored as correct if a female first name plus a last name other than the subject's last name is given.

Question 10 requires that the entire series must be performed correctly in order to be scored as correct. Any error in the series or unwillingness to attempt the series is scored as incorrect.

SCORING OF THE SPMSQ

The data suggest that both education and race influence performance on the SPMSQ, and they must be taken into account in evaluating the score attained by an individual.

For purposes of scoring, three educational levels have been established: (a) persons who have had only a grade school education; (b) persons who have had any high school education or who have completed high school; and (c) persons who have had any education beyond the high school level, including college, graduate school, or business school.

For white subjects with at least some high school education, but not more than high school education, the following criteria have been established:

0–2 ERRORS	INTACT INTELLECTUAL FUNCTIONING
3–4 ERRORS	MILD INTELLECTUAL IMPAIRMENT
5–7 ERRORS	MODERATE INTELLECTUAL IMPAIRMENT
8–10 ERRORS	SEVERE INTELLECTUAL IMPAIRMENT

Allow one more error if subject has had only a grade school education.

Allow one less error if subject has had education beyond high school.

Allow one more error for black subjects, using identical education criteria.

Source: Reprinted with permission from E. Pfeiffer, A Short Portable Mental Status Questionnaire for the Assessment of Organic Brain Deficit in Elderly Patients, *JAGS,* Vol. 23, No. 10, pp. 433–441, © 1975, Williams & Wilkins.

Questions included in the Mini-Mental State Examination and SPMSQ that are typical of any mental status screening examination are (1) personal data such as name, address, and telephone number; (2) orientation to time of day, month, and year; (3) serial reversals, spelling a word backward, or counting backward; and (4) recalling several objects after a period of time. Other items in a mental screening test may include naming objects or body parts, drawing or copying figures, and discussing current events. In most instances, inability to respond correctly to more than two or three questions indicates the need for additional testing. Failure on screening does not automatically indicate the presence of dementia; further testing is needed to confirm this diagnosis.

Neurological Evaluation

When considering changes identified in the neurological evaluation, one must remember that neurological examination of the elderly tends to show considerable differences when compared to that of a younger population. Most of the changes seen in the elderly are related to the peripheral organs rather than to actual changes in the central nervous system. One of the most important aspects of the neurological examination is the ability of certain items to differentiate between Alzheimer's disease and other disorders that may present as Alzheimer's disease. For example, neurological changes such as cerebellar ataxia and involuntary movements noted early in the dementing disease may indicate Creutzfeldt-Jakob disease; focal neurological signs, such as weakness on one side or visual field defects, are distinguishing features of multi-infarct dementia.

In advanced cases of Alzheimer's disease the neurological abnormalities are specific as opposed to diffuse, particularly in changes of gait, posture, and reflexes (Paulson, 1977). In early cases the neurological examination frequently shows no significant change or abnormalities. Changes are noted only on comparison of examinations over time.

Laboratory Tests

The purpose of laboratory tests is to rule out pre-existing conditions that could affect physical and mental health. The complete blood count detects anemia and infections. An analysis of the blood chemistry helps to rule out conditions such as kidney or liver malfunctions or unsuspected diabetes. Vitamin deficiencies can also be detected through blood chemistry analysis. Vitamin deficiency caused by malnutrition or poor nutrition is a reversible cause of dementia. Although thyroid problems identifiable by blood work are among the more common reversible causes of dementia in the elderly (Mace & Rabins, 1981), thyroid studies are not part of routine laboratory tests.

An article by Recer (1996) reports the possible development of a laboratory test of blood and skin cells for early detection of the disease. The article quotes Dr. Jay H. Robbins, a National Cancer Institute researcher who led the team that developed the test. Dr. Robbins states "This test could be useful in identifying the disease absolutely in patients who are diagnosed as probable Alzheimer's disease" (p. A–2). At this time, however, the test is not on the market.

Lumbar Puncture

Lumbar puncture, also known as a spinal tap, is performed to rule out the presence of abnormal proteins in the spinal fluid. It is helpful in excluding chronic infections such as meningitis, tuberculosis, syphilis, and the like. Unless there is reason to suspect a specific disorder, this test is not routinely done.

Electroencephalogram

The electroencephalogram (EEG) records the electrical activity of the brain. Changes in EEG have been noted in some normal elderly persons. The most common change is a slight slowing of the alpha rhythm (Hughes & Cayaffa, 1977). In normal aging, however, pronounced general slowing of the brain waves is not common.

Early-stage Alzheimer's clients may show normal EEG patterns. Nevertheless, as the disease progresses there will be an eventual progressive slowing and disorganization of the background pattern. Alpha activity is reduced and finally disappears. Because there are no EEG changes specific to Alzheimer's disease, a diagnosis cannot be made solely on the basis of such changes.

Computed Axial Tomography (CT)

Unlike x-ray studies, the CT scan is able to visualize soft tissue. The introduction of the CT scan in the 1970s made it easier to perform evaluations of cerebral structures in vivo. It also made it easier to establish brain and behavior relationships.

The most widely used method of evaluating CT scan data consists of evaluating the size of the cerebral ventricles and sulci. Although some studies have found some relationship between the CT imaging data and the level of cognitive functioning (Naeser et al., 1980; Yamaura et al., 1980), many individuals with dementia have been shown to have no obvious cerebral "atrophy" and others with marked "atrophy" have no dementia (Boller et al., 1980). To date, the greatest value of the CT scan in evaluating dementia clients has been its ability to identify other disorders such as subdural hematoma, brain tumor, hydrocephalus, and dementia associated with vascular disease (McKhann et al., 1984).

Positron Emission Tomography

Positron emission tomography (PET) has been used as a research tool to study changes in brain metabolism and regional cerebral blood flow. The PET scan, like the CT scan, makes use of an imaging device and constructs tomographic images of the brain by means of a computer. The major difference between the two is that PET images represent regional brain function, whereas CT images represent regional brain structures. PET scans allow quantitative assessment of the rate of glucose utilization, oxygen consumption, and regional cerebral blood flow.

Elderly persons without central nervous disorders do not, as a rule, show significantly decreased cerebral blood flow. A reduction in cerebral blood flow has been observed in all dementias and in depression (Mathew et al., 1980). Individuals with multi-infarct dementia show a reduction in cerebral blood flow in areas that correspond to the history and clinical localization of the infarcts.

PET scans of persons with Alzheimer's disease tend to show a common trajectory. In the earlier stages there appears to be a lessening of activity on one side or the other of the neocortex in the parietal region. Over time PET scans can track a systematic decrease in brain activity from the crown, spreading downward and then frontward toward the temporal cortex where the hippocampus lies. From this point damage appears to move to the prefrontal cortex. Since current PET studies reveal a significant variation even among normal subjects, changes may have to be severe to be detected (McKhann et al., 1984). PET scans are not always available or used routinely in evaluation for Alzheimer's disease.

Magnetic Resonance Imaging

Magnetic resonance imaging (MRI) uses no radiation to produce its image. Because of the public's perception of the term "nuclear" as having to do with radioactivity, the term nuclear magnetic resonance was altered to magnetic resonance imaging, or MRI. A primary part of the MRI apparatus is a cylinder-shaped electromagnet. Unlike other tools, MRI reveals the demarcation of gray and white matter of the brain. It is useful in studies of demyelinating disorders and as a research tool in dementia since the MRI appears to be able to pick up early atrophy in the hippocampus of people who go on to develop Alzheimer's disease.

Neuropsychological Assessment

By definition, individuals with dementia have impaired intellectual function. Studies have shown that demented individuals do not perform as well on standardized intelligence tests as normal control groups (Miller, 1981). Standardized intelligence tests do not provide sufficient information regarding the nature of the intellectual deficits seen in different dementia syndromes, however. The report of the NINCDS-ADRDA work group (McKhann et al., 1984) suggests that cognitive processes evaluated in Alzheimer's disease should be done by means of a carefully selected neuropsychological test battery that measures specific abilities such as memory.

Impaired memory, one of the hallmarks of dementia, is frequently reported as an early sign of Alzheimer's disease. It often remains the most conspicuous defect during the first stage of the disease. The impairment is global in nature and involves both short- and long-term memory in all modalities. As the disease progresses, memory impairment gradually broadens and merges into a more global intellectual impairment.

A frequent question regarding memory and dementia is "Why do people with dementia remember what happened many years earlier?" Investigations by Sanders and Warrington (1971) and others (Miller, l981) suggest that, despite the impression that remote memory is preserved, it too is impaired. Other areas of cognitive functioning affected by Alzheimer's disease include orientation, language skills, praxis, attention, visual perception, problem solving skills, and social function. Neuropsychological testing is needed to determine which areas are affected and to what degree they are affected.

Because there are no normative population standards for many of these tests, abnormal performance can be determined only by comparison with a normal control group matched for age, sex, and local education. "Normal" in this instance refers to subjects who are functioning independently within the community and who do not have any history of psychiatric problems. A score falling in the lowest fifth percentile of an individual's "normal" control group may be designated "abnormal" (McKhann et al., 1984). Repeated testing with the same measures can be used to document progression of the disease.

Confirmation of dementia by a neuropsychological test should be based on "measurable abnormalities in two or more aspects of cognition" (McKhann et al., 1984, p. 941). The particular battery of neuropsychological tests is currently left to the discretion of the neuropsychologist.

Making the Diagnosis

There is a twofold purpose in seeking the evaluation outlined above: first, to determine whether dementia is present, and second, to identify causative factors. At the present there is no single uniform profile of an Alzheimer's patient that can be measured by testing.

Test results will vary from patient to patient, depending on the patient's age, previous medical and mental status, educational level, and the stage of the disease at which he or she has finally sought a diagnosis. Not all dementia clients seek a diagnosis in the early stages. Many do not seek help or information until they can no longer function without intervention. Approximately 10% of those persons seeking an evaluation for dementia will, on evaluation, prove to have some type of disorder not related to Alzheimer's disease.

Despite the development of sophisticated tools such as PET and MRI, there is no single positive test for Alzheimer's disease on the market. Compounding this problem is the fact that the earlier one tries to detect the disease, the more difficult it is to diagnose. In the early stages of the disease, a CT scan, an EEG, and other physiological tests will probably be negative. In the case of a well-educated individual, screening on a mental status examination may also prove negative in the very early stages.

Yet early detection is important for client and family. Identifying the disease in its earliest stages helps to establish a baseline that can be used for comparison with later evaluations to measure changes, and offers the client and family a chance to mobilize their resources and to work toward managing the future.

Progressive worsening of cognitive function over time without change in other areas indicates the presence of dementia and could signal the need to intervene in cases where the individual may be a hazard in the workplace, such as an airplane pilot who cannot fly safely or a physician who confuses drugs. "Over time," however, may mean anywhere from 6 months to 1 year or more. In the later stages, changes will be noted in mental status and on neuropsychological testing. Finally, changes will be noted in all the procedures discussed earlier.

Thus the current diagnosis of Alzheimer's disease relies heavily on case history, changes in cognitive functioning over time, and the absence of other causative factors. Dementia can be determined on the basis of changes in cognitive functioning, but Alzheimer's disease is determined only after other causative factors of dementia have been eliminated. On the basis of the clinical tests, the physician will rule out the possibility of reversible causes of dementia such as drug toxicity, metabolic diseases, infection, and so on. The next step is to rule out irreversible causes such as ischemia (in multi-infarct dementia and cerebrovascular accident), disorders of the extrapyramidal system (in Huntington's and Parkinson's diseases), depression, hydrocephalus, and chronic states of confusion. Table 2–1 compares the onset and distinguishing features in Alzheimer's disease with normal forgetfulness due to aging, depression, chronic schizophrenia, multi-infarct dementia, and delirium, which must be considered in the differential diagnosis of Alzheimer's disease.

About 10% of the individuals tested will have a treatable condition. The remaining 90% will be diagnosed as having irreversible dementia. Of those having irreversible dementia, approximately 50% will have dementia of the Alzheimer's type, 30% will have multi-infarct dementia, and the remaining 20% will have other types of irreversible dementia such as Pick's disease. When all other possibilities have been ruled out, the physician will offer a diagnosis of Alzheimer's disease.

BEHAVIORAL CHANGES IN ALZHEIMER'S DISEASE

Before proceeding to a discussion of the "four stages" of dementia, it will be useful to review three systems of behavioral staging of Alzheimer's disease prepared by individuals in three different settings: (1) clinical social work and teaching, (2) family support, and (3) clinical research psychiatry.

Clinical Social Work and Teaching

Gwyther and Matteson (1983) describe three behavioral stages of Alzheimer's disease: the early, middle, and final stages. In the early stage, which may last for 2 to 4 years, changes in memory and behavior are subtle. The family may refuse to recognize the implications of the changes, but as the disease progresses the individual's performance at work falls off.

In the middle stage there is progressive memory loss, aphasia, agnosia, apraxia, wandering, and repetitive movements such as tapping. Changes in eating habits may also be noticed. This stage lasts longer than either of the other two stages. In Gwyther and Matteson's system the diagnosis is usually made during this stage.

The final stage, according to these investigators, is generally short. Clients do not eat or communicate, they may be incontinent, and they may have grand mal seizures. Total personal care is required, and the person with Alzheimer's disease may not be able to recognize the caregiver. It is during this stage that families must face the possibility of the patient's institutionalization.

Table 2–1 Comparison of Features Associated with Dementias

	Slow Onset	Reduced Level of Consciousness	Progression of Symptoms	Memory Loss	Cognitive Impairment	Emotional Incontinence*	Vegetative Symptoms#	Paranoia Hallucinations
Normal Age-Related Decline	yes	no	none	mild	no	no	no	no
Alzheimer's Disease	yes	no	slow	yes	yes	yes	yes	yes
Multi-Infarct Dementia	no	no	step-wise	yes	yes	yes	varies	varies
Depression	no	no	rapid	no	no	no	yes	no
Delirium	no	yes	fluctuates	yes	yes	yes	yes	yes
Chronic Schizophrenia	yes	no	may be episodic	no	yes	yes	varies	yes

*Inappropriate or sudden crying or laughing for no apparent reason.
#Vegetative symptoms include changes in the sleep-wake cycle, loss of appetite, and excessive eating.

Family Support

Morscheck (1984) suggests that there are four behavioral stages, with stage three representing an intensification of the symptoms in stage two. Memory undergoes extreme deterioration, language deteriorates over time, agitation and energy levels increase, sleep disturbances occur, and total personal care is eventually needed.

Clinical Research Psychiatry

In the Global Deterioration Scale (GDS) for Age-Associated Cognitive and Alzheimer's Disease, Reisberg, Ferris, and Crook (1983) present a seven-point scale that includes behavioral descriptions and psychometric concomitants to determine clinically the severity of dementia exhibited by the individual. Determination of an individual's stage and placement on the scale is made via observed clinical characteristics and test scores. The behavioral descriptions offered by these investigators under "clinical characteristics" may be likened to the "stages" observed by Morscheck and Gwyther.

Of the behavioral views outlined above, Gwyther and Matteson's is the simplest for families to understand and Reisberg's offers the most precise description of symptomatology along with psychometric concomitants for professionals who may need a more exacting guide for diagnosing and documenting the progression of the client's behavioral changes.

Four-Stage Alzheimer's Scale for Therapists

The importance of stages or identifiable landmarks should not be underestimated when working with dementia clients and their families. All parties need concrete information to help them recognize where they are in relation to the progression of the disease. This four-stage scale of the progression of the disease is similar to those used by Gwyther and Matteson and by Morscheck when describing the symptoms and progression of the disease as observed by the family. It has proved helpful when developing strategies to be used during therapy sessions.

Stage 1

- Duration: 2 to 4 years.
- General features: Client is physically and socially intact; families may not recognize implications of what appear to be minor deficits.
- Symptoms: Lack of initiative, overreaction to events, memory loss, lack of spontaneity, feelings of losing control, hostile behavior.
- Speech and language: Anomia, reduced comprehension, reduced information content, reduced attention, frequent requests for repetition, mild agnosia or apraxia evidenced by patient or family reports of difficulty reading or seeing or problems managing articles of clothing (such as tying a necktie) (see Figure 2–1).

In stage 1 the individual is physically intact and cannot be differentiated from normal individuals on the basis of physical appearance. In this stage, the individual functions through a primary resource or caregiver. It is not uncommon to find a husband or wife responding for the affected person. For example, when one client was asked to describe when he first noticed that he was having problems, his wife responded "You remember, Steve, you couldn't tie your tie." In the workplace, coworkers may have to pick up part of the individual's work load. The client shows a lack of initiative to start new projects and

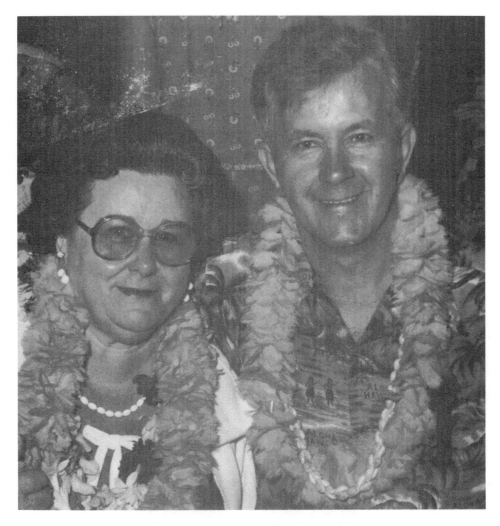

Figure 2–1 Stage 1. The client is physically and socially intact. This man looks well. At this stage, the family may not recognize implications of what appear to be minor deficits.

begins to rely on others to cover up the loss in memory. For example, the husband may take over the wife's job of making up the shopping list.

Stage 2

- Duration: 4 years (average).
- General features: Loss of social ability, sleeping disorders, communication difficulties, appearance of seizures, difficulties in ADLs.
- Symptoms: Progressive memory loss, hallucinations, hostility, paranoia, excessive passivity, lability, wandering.

- Speech and language: The client will retain some ability to repeat information. There is increased anomia evidenced by difficulty in naming objects, paraphasia (e.g., substitution of inappropriate words in a sentence or in connected speech), concrete concept formation evidenced by literal interpretation of all stimuli, impaired writing and number concepts, impaired comprehension, ideational apraxia (e.g., difficulty completing a task such as lighting a match), and agnosia. Client will retain some ability to repeat information.

Sometime during stage 2 (Figure 2–2), families that have not sought help earlier now do so because the loss in all areas can no longer be ignored. In this stage, individuals who are still employed rely heavily on others (such as a secretary) to carry the work load. Some individuals may relive old grudges, believe there are intruders in the house, or forget to turn off the stove. Some become excessively passive; others become hostile. Lability is not uncommon. By the middle of stage 2 individuals will no longer be able to remain employed, and the homemaker will need help at home.

Stage 3

- Duration: 2 to 4 years.
- General features: Progressive loss of mental abilities, susceptibility to illness and infection, flattened affect, mild to moderate physical problems that become progressively more serious.
- Symptoms: Overeating, hyper- or hypoactivity, incontinence, severe communication deficits, increase in seizure activity.
- Speech and language: Echolalia, repetition of words and phrases of others; palilalia, also called autoecholalia, where the individual repeats part of his or her own sentences in ongoing speech; dysarthria, slurred speech due to motor dysfunction; jargon, meaningless utterances; visual agnosia,

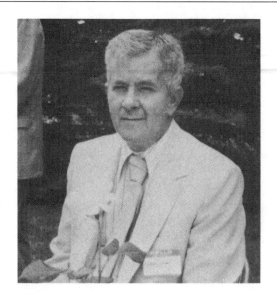

Figure 2–2 Stage 2. The physical changes shown here may be too subtle for the outsider to notice. Family members, however, pointed to a "dullness" or "lack of sparkle," particularly in the client's eyes. At this stage the client could not function without the aid of his caregiver.

difficulty or inability to interpret visual stimuli in the absence of significant visual impairment; poor attention; poor engagement; severely reduced comprehension; and latent, delayed response.

In stage 3 (Figure 2–3), physical changes that began in stage 2 are now obvious. There is a change in gait and facial expression, and responses are slow. The individual may talk to inanimate objects or reflections in a mirror or window. The individual has difficulty in separating reality from fantasy, and some individuals believe that actions seen on television are actually occurring. The symptom of overeating does not mean that the individual will gain weight. Frequently there is a change in the individual's metabolism and a weight loss. The appearance of incontinence seems to be one of the most difficult problems for family members to cope with. Families often begin seriously to consider placing the individual in a nursing home when incontinence becomes a problem, but the same conditions that make home care hard to manage—hostility, incontinence, and feeding problems—may make nursing home placement difficult.

Stage 4

- Duration: Uncertain. Clients have been known to remain in the final stage of the disease well beyond 2 years, whereas others die within 6 months.
- General features: Severe physical and mental deterioration.
- Symptoms: Inability to eat, loss of voluntary movements, regression to fetal stage, respiratory problems, changes in auto-immune function.
- Speech and language: Eventual total loss of all communication skills.

In stage 4 of Alzheimer's disease (Figure 2–4), there are noticeable changes in EEG, and PET and CT scans. Among the symptoms, the inability to eat is a primary concern in this last stage of Alzheimer's disease; it is listed under symptoms rather than speech/language because it is not a true

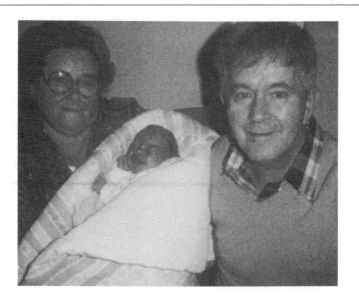

Figure 2–3 Stage 3. People outside the family circle now note the change in the facial expression. The client's affect has flattened and, as one person said, "life has gone out of his eyes."

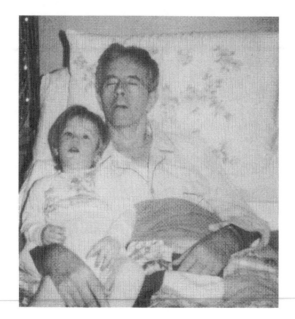

Figure 2–4 Stage 4. This picture leaves little doubt as to the devastating toll the disease has taken. The client is no longer ambulatory, is incontinent, and has difficulty eating.

dysphagia. Although the Alzheimer's client is unable to swallow food, there does not appear to be any difficulty swallowing saliva, and even terminal individuals can remain supine without aspirating. Ultimately the body's immune system breaks down, and death is the final outcome.

As the disease progresses through these four stages, the therapist and the family shift their emphasis from cognitive to physical concerns. In the early stages, client needs focus on memory, socialization, and maintaining a daily routine. In the later stages, emphasis shifts to basic ADLs such as toileting, eating, and maintaining contact with a significant other. Regardless of what stage the client is in, families need professional help in learning how to deal with the disease.

When reviewing these stages, it is important to keep several points in mind. First, the symptoms presented may be attributed to any of a number of different causative factors that need to be evaluated. Second, none of the symptoms is written in stone, since not all symptoms of the disease will be exhibited in each client. Third, although most symptoms will continue to manifest as the disease progresses, some will disappear. Fourth, the disease can last for more than a decade. A summary of the four stages is given in Table 2–2.

Table 2–2 Summary of the Four Stages of Alzheimer's Disease

Stage	Features	Duration (Years)
1	Physically and socially intact	2–4
2	Loss of social ability	~4
3	Progressive loss of mental and physical abilities	2–4
4	Severe physical and mental deterioration	Uncertain

Management

FAMILY NEEDS

Rabins (1984) distinguishes between the role changes and the responsibility changes that Alzheimer's disease often imposes on family members. According to Rabins, roles are a reflection of social positions within a given network, and responsibilities are tasks that an individual performs. Frequently it is easier to make adjustments in responsibilities than in roles.

The needs of the members of the family as well as their roles change as the affected individual's condition grows worse (Gwyther, 1985). In the initial stage of the disease, family members may erratically embrace self-help or cure-seeking solutions. They ask the client to "try harder," and then they feel angry as well as guilty when the client fails. Family conflicts may arise when several family members have differing views of what course should be taken.

As the disease progresses, the demands on the family increase. Family members may suffer from isolation, anger, guilt, and lack of privacy, as well as a sense of loss. In addition, the physical demands on the primary caregiver may begin to take a toll. Persons with Alzheimer's disease who have sleep disorders or who wander can be a particular problem for the caregiver, who is unable to find respite.

In the final stages of the disease, families are most concerned with decisions regarding nursing home versus home-care. Families frequently suffer a mixture of guilt, anger, and frustration. Their financial reality may not allow for the type of care that the caregiver would like to provide. Horror stories about nursing homes and encounters with indifferent professionals cause some families to deny the need for help until the caregiver encounters a medical crisis.

In each stage of the disease, the caregiver is as much a client in need of help as the Alzheimer's client. The overriding feelings expressed by family members are helplessness and loss of control. They cannot do anything about the course of the disease, they cannot direct the services they receive, and often they can no longer control their own lives because of the demands of caregiving. One of the primary needs of family members, therefore, is support. The support group helps family members to know that they are not alone. ADRDA, with chapters all over the United States, has been successful in directing the energies of Alzheimer's disease caregivers into a constructive force in education, research, and advocacy.

Family members share their experiences and discuss ways of obtaining needed services. They learn about the disease and work toward a common goal. Some hospitals and nursing homes are now offering support through individual counseling by a social worker or in group sessions.

Respite also ranks high among family needs. In response to this need, adult day care programs have become more available. Some nursing homes offer 3-day-weekend stays to Alzheimer's clients whose care-givers need time for themselves. Above all, the caregiver needs to feel in control of his or her situation.

CASE MANAGEMENT FOR THE ALZHEIMER'S CLIENT

To work effectively with a client, it is often helpful to have some understanding of the client's needs that go beyond the specific clinical setting. In addition to traditional forms of clinical case management offered by any institution, clients may avail themselves of other case management programs that may act independently of the institution. The primary objective of these management programs is to coordinate, and to help the family and Alzheimer's client obtain, needed services. The focus of these programs is the family (caregiver) as the decision maker and the Alzheimer's client as the passive receiver of services designed to help the family cope.

Working with the Entire Family

Alzheimer's disease is a family problem. It affects the lives of the Alzheimer's person, the primary caregiver, and all family members. Effective case management must consider the needs of all those involved. Although the needs of each member of the family will differ, supportive therapy alone is not sufficient. According to Wasow (1986), "The focus has been on the individual caregiver, rather than on the caregiver as part of three different family systems: the family of origin, family of procreation, the spouse's family of origin, and [how] the characteristics of each may affect caregiving help, attitudes, behaviors, and experiences" (p. 96).

A family's feelings of helplessness are frequently mixed with feelings of anger and suspicion directed toward a system of health care that they view as being inadequate, uncaring, and self-serving. Case management programs have been beneficial to many Alzheimer's families in assisting them to gain access to the system with minimal distress. Successful case management programs have looked toward reducing family feelings of stress by including family members as part of the decision-making team.

Independent Case Management Programs

Case management is not a new concept. All health care providers perform case management activities. The concept of the case manager independent of the providing agency or service is relatively new, however (President's Commission on Mental Health, 1978). Today, case management is recognized as an essential method of overcoming the complexity and fragmentation of health service systems and reaching an inadequately serviced population (Miller, 1983). Case management may be provided on either a short- or long-term basis and is sometimes referred to as service management, case coordination, or resource coordination (Steinberg, 1985). Case management programs vary greatly in degree of control and scope of services provided to clients.

Some programs cover all aspects of information, referral, assessment, service purchase, service delivery, and service monitoring. Other programs, such as the one presented here, are limited to information, referral, and service monitoring. Comprehensive services have the advantage of purchasing services from competing institutions. The case manager in such programs can help to provide needed services more efficiently and at a greater cost-to-benefit ratio than clients could achieve on their own. Clients may find this type of service advantageous not only because of the dollars and cents involved but because of the concept of "one-stop shopping" with a service whose vested interest is in the clients.

Ross, Riffer, and Switalski (1983) describe the functions of the case manager in terms of eight roles: facilitator, linker, supporter, broker, monitor, bridger, catalyst, and advocate. The manager acts as a facilitator in helping the client interact with the system and as a linker by bringing clients and services together. The manager is a supporter by showing concern for and confidence in the client's abilities. Service purchase and follow up puts the manager in the roles of broker and monitor. As a bridger and catalyst, the manager finds gaps in services and communications between client and service agencies and brings problems to the attention of others to facilitate change. Finally, as an advocate, the manager assists the clients in protecting their rights.

Comprehensive Case Management

Ideally, a comprehensive case management program should be able to match a client with a needed service and to provide ongoing monitoring and reassessment of the client's needs to make service adjustments. The comprehensive system includes assessment, referral, monitoring, service purchase, and service delivery.

In a comprehensive case management program, once an appointment has been made through the intake person a case manager is assigned. The case manager is responsible for all aspects of service to the client and acts as the contact person for the client when additional service is requested or when a complaint is lodged. Although the word "client" is used to mean the Alzheimer's patient, it is the caregiver acting on the client's behalf who is the decision maker working with the case manager. Hereafter, the word "client" will encompass both the patient and the caregiver.

Assessment. At the outset the case manager assesses the client's needs. This may be done by a registered nurse in the client's home or at an assessment center. The Alzheimer's patient and the caregiver are interviewed. There is also an assessment of the patient's ADLs and an evaluation of the client's home environment. Depending on the service provider, there may be a complete financial review. The assessment is a critical first step in matching client needs and appropriate service.

Case planning. The next step for the case manager is case planning. The three steps in case planning are (1) to list the problems identified in the assessment; (2) to determine the necessary, immediate, and primary goals; and (3) to list the steps that need to be taken to solve each problem. As part of the case planning, the case manager determines which services are available, approximately how long they will be needed, their cost, and whether or not they are acceptable to the client. The case manager must also determine the appropriate care setting. For example, some services can be provided in the home of the client, whereas others may require an institutional setting.

The types of services needed by the Alzheimer's client generally fall into one of three categories: social support, health support, and information and referral. Social supports are those services needed to maintain the individual (at home or in an institution) that do not directly affect the individual's health status. These include homemaker services, transportation, Meals on Wheels, and inclusion in support groups. Many of the social supports needed to maintain the Alzheimer's client are designed to aid the caregiver as well. Health supports are those services needed to maintain the individual's physical well-being. In addition to physician services, respite, health screening, and pharmaceutical services are included under health support. Those services not provided by the particular agency in charge of the individual's case management fall into the category of information and referral. Services concerning resource counseling, ombudsman, and legal problems generally fall into this category.

Once services are arranged, it is the responsibility of the case manager to maintain contact with the client, to monitor the services being provided, and to assess periodically service needs.

Current trends in aging and an increasing need for services have given rise to assessment centers for older individuals. Some senior citizen centers, under the support of state governments, also offer comprehensive case management for elderly adults. Comprehensive assessment and case management services for Alzheimer's clients are currently available at a number of institutions. Information regarding what is available in a particular area can be obtained by calling or writing for information to the ADRDA.

Selective Case Management

An alternative type of case management, which since 1981 has been provided by the author to clients seeking assistance, is much narrower in scope and provides as much or as little assistance as the client requests. The objective is to place the family members in control of the situation by helping them determine a plan of action that includes all areas of client needs. The case manager assists in matching the client and the service by offering the client a choice of service providers. By aiding the family members in determining a course of action that they can implement, feelings of helplessness are reduced, thus relieving stress and allowing the family to act in a positive manner.

Family members are seen together. Typically, one member of the family calls for an appointment and arranges to have all family members gather at one place for the meeting. It is not uncommon to find three adult children and their spouses each with varying degrees of information and differences of opinions ready to tell the primary caregiver what to do. Despite initial differences of opinions, family members who call for appointments want help and are usually willing to work together for a common goal once that goal is identified. Indeed, the first job of the case manager is to help the family members recognize their common goal.

Regardless of what stage the Alzheimer's client has reached, families need information and review in the following six areas: (1) medical, (2) financial, (3) legal, (4) home care, (5) institutional placement, and (6) therapy. Therapy is placed last on the list because a family must understand the situation in the first five areas before they are ready to consider therapy of any type. Once these areas are reviewed, a plan of action can be established.

Medical. Families need to discuss with each other and with a knowledgeable person what Alzheimer's disease is and how it will affect their lives. They need to be certain that the client has had adequate medical and psychological evaluation. They must be assured that the client is receiving the best, most up-to-date treatment available. In some instances families want to know about current research problems. They also want to know about genetic findings and the probability of other family members developing the disease.

Financial. Long-term care can leave families without financial resources. Adult children are concerned that they may be legally liable for the care of their parents. Older women may be left with no financial support if their husbands' pensions must go to pay for nursing home care. Family members must decide who can contribute financially to the patient's care. Before a decision can be reached, there must be a realistic estimate of current and future needs. There must also be an understanding of state regulations regarding financial responsibility for medical and other services, as well as what constitutes personal and estate property that must be used for the client's care.

Legal. Most individuals assume that they have the right to make decisions concerning life and death and to handle all finances for immediate relatives such as a spouse or parent. In a family where there is no question regarding care or responsibility, decisions may be made by a single individual. In most instances, families look to the primary caregiver to make the decisions and to sign documents for treatment and payment. This is not always the case, however. Legally, unless an individual has specific powers of attorney or guardianship of both person and estate, the right to make decisions may be subject to debate.

Consider, for example, the situation in which an Alzheimer's patient in a nursing home is no longer eating and a decision must be made about whether or not to insert a feeding tube. The patient's wife tells the nursing home that she will not authorize a gastrostomy because she would like her husband to be allowed to die in peace. The patient's daughter, however, feels that she could not bear to watch her father starve to death and goes to court to gain guardianship and to force the nursing home to have the gastrostomy tube inserted. When families are not aware of problems that may arise and legal steps that must be taken to avoid conflict, permanent damage can be done to the family system.

Home care. Many families are unaware of what type of home care assistance is available in their area and how assistance is funded. Caregivers need information about programs such as Meals on Wheels, senior shopping services, and chore-worker services. Not all areas have services that are readily available, but families should know what they need, where to find it, and how much it costs.

Institutional placement. At the onset of a disease such as Alzheimer's, families often vow that they will never institutionalize an ill member. In most instances, however, wonderful intentions and resolve are forced to give way to necessity. Eventually, the Alzheimer's client will no longer be able to leave home to attend day care or for short-term respite care. The client will become incontinent, and physical debilitation will require increased attention. When this occurs, many caregivers find it necessary to seek placement in either a personal care home (assisted living) or a nursing home.

Families must understand the difference between the personal care home, which cannot accommodate nonambulatory clients in need of medical services, and the nursing home, which has several different levels of care ranging from skilled nursing care to custodial care. Families also need to know which facilities can care for the patient and the costs of that care.

Therapy. For many families therapy is the last consideration. Some tend to be too overwhelmed with day-to-day demands to consider therapy either for themselves or for the Alzheimer's client. Most never consider therapy for the Alzheimer's client because they are told that nothing can be done or because they know the disease cannot be stopped.

Despite the negative prognosis inherent in Alzheimer's disease, family members express a need to "do something" for the Alzheimer's client. When therapy is offered as a partnership arrangement to help ease the burden and to assist the client to function at the highest level feasible, many family members are willing to try. In the early stages, when cooperation of the Alzheimer's client is readily obtainable, therapy offers both parties a chance to work together to improve their quality of life. Therapy can play an important role in alleviating the long-term burden of the caregiver and in helping Alzheimer's clients to function at their optimal level (see Part II).

The plan of action. After all the options open to the family in the areas outlined above are discussed, a plan of action is developed. First, problem areas are listed individually with possible solutions. For each area where services are needed, the family members are offered the names and telephone numbers of up to three agencies or service providers for that particular area of need. Next, the family members are given information about the progressive stages of Alzheimer's disease and about services that may be needed in the future. Finally, family members are given suggestions about what to look for when choosing a service and questions to ask the potential provider. Family members are encouraged to make their own contact with the service provider and to follow through on service. If for any reason the family members are not satisfied with the service provided, additional agencies (if available) are offered. In the event that family members request additional services, such as service monitoring, the case manager must decide what services he or she will provide.

The two systems of case management discussed have distinct advantages. The major advantage of the first system is "one-stop shopping" and the possibility of having the services of the case manager covered by some type of funding. Although the second system offers only selective services and is not covered by third-party payment, it provides an opportunity for individual family members to have more central control over their situation since information about available services and a plan of action for the future are provided for their personal use. They also have the advantage of a service whose sole interest is client satisfaction.

Part II

FUNCTIONAL ASSESSMENTS AND INTERVENTIONS FOR DEMENTIA CLIENTS

Language Considerations in Alzheimer's Disease

How well we communicate depends primarily on our ability to use language. Any reduction in language, or the ability to manipulate language, reduces our ability to maintain contact with others. In Alzheimer's disease, the loss of communication skills affects the individual suffering the loss as well as the support network of that individual. Therefore, increasing and enhancing communication between the Alzheimer's client and everyone with whom he or she comes into contact should be a priority.

Bayles and Kaszniak state "The clinician testing the dementia patient should be concerned with evaluating communication rather than knowledge of language per se" (1991, p. 161). Their rationale behind this statement lies in the dementia patient's relatively preserved linguistic skills in the presence of decreased communicative ability. Nevertheless, differential diagnosis of preserved and disordered language is a vital part of the diagnostic process. The literature on language changes in Alzheimer's disease is sparse. In *Principles of Neurology* (1977), Adams and Victor describe speech in Alzheimer's clients as halting, with the client unable to think of specific words. Similar problems are noted in writing. The therapist sometimes cannot determine whether the Alzheimer's client does not understand a complex command or does understand but immediately forgets (Miller, 1981). Some observers describe the speech of the Alzheimer's client as fluent and with preserved syntax; others describe speech in later stages as bizarre, with little communicative intent (Obler & Albert, 1981). Mentis, Briggs-Whittaker, and Gramigna (1995) found that Alzheimer's subjects showed a reduced ability to change topics, difficulty in actively contributing to propositional development of a topic, and failure to consistently maintain a topic in a clear and coherent manner. On the other hand, the flow of discourse was preserved.

Although, with few exceptions, individuals with dementia do not show the classic symptoms of aphasia that are found in persons with focal brain lesions (Wechsler, 1977), aphasia, apraxia, and agnosia are part of the dementia syndrome. Aphasia refers to an acquired disorder of the ability to use the conventional symbols of language, reflected in altered speech, writing, reading, and mathematical tasks. Agnosia refers to an acquired cortical sensory or perceptual disorder, and apraxia refers to an impairment of the ability to carry out sequential voluntary movements in the absence of obvious sensorimotor deficits.

Part of the frustration in attempting to classify and categorize language disturbances in Alzheimer's disease is the variation of symptoms among persons having the disease (Obler, 1983). Nevertheless, language and language-related difficulties are common in all stages of dementia. Naming difficulty is perhaps the most frequently mentioned language sign associated with dementia. Rochford (1971) and Barker and Lawson (1968) found that naming disorders differ in persons with dementia and those with classical aphasia due to stroke. The aphasic person generally knows the object that is misidentified, whereas the demented person misidentifies because the object itself is unknown. Naming performance improves in demented individuals when object identification difficulty is minimized. The aphasic individual does not show this type of improvement. Bayles and Kaszniak (1991) state that "Differentiating the aphasia patient from the dementia patient may not be as simple as previously believed, because some aphasia patients demonstrate cognitive impairment and some dementia patients exhibit language impairment disproportionate to their cognitive functioning" (p. 201). It is certainly more likely that patients with Wernicke's (fluent) aphasias and preserved repetition are more likely to be confused with dementia patients than patients with Broca's aphasia. To differentiate aphasia due to focal brain damage from dementia, Bayles and Kaszniak (1991) recommend testing verbal and nonverbal memory, visuospatial construction, orientation, and linguistic reasoning, as well as fluency, auditory comprehension, repetition, reading, writing, praxis, naming, and spontaneous language.

Albert and colleagues (1981) summarize the language deficits of dementia as

1. incoherent output due to a breakdown in logical associations of speech
2. naming difficulties due to a reduction in vocabulary
3. simplification of syntax
4. perseveration (intrusive speech)
5. echolalia
6. introduction of improbable or unlikely phrases
7. circumlocution
8. an increase in the above deficits as the length of conversation increases

Although these investigators also reported the presence of comprehension difficulties, they believe it is possible that such difficulties may be due to a generalized intellectual deficit and are not specifically language related.

Apraxia becomes apparent when the Alzheimer's client is asked to perform a series of acts in sequence to achieve a given goal, such as picking up and lighting a match (Heilman, 1979). When testing for apraxia, it is difficult to know whether the individual is truly apraxic or has simply forgotten the goal. Visually, individuals appear to have difficulty with object identification. Studies by Ernst and coworkers (1970b) and Willanger and Klee (1966) reported perceptual distortions during fixation and disorders of a gnostic and praxic nature in a small percentage of dementia patients.

The course of speech and language deterioration in Alzheimer's disease has been described by a number of investigators (Obler, 1979; 1983; Beasley & Davis, 1981). In the early stages there is a noticeable use of vague terms and word-finding difficulty. Perseverative or intrusive speech is apparent. As the disease progresses there is an increase of intrusive speech in the form of palilalia (sometimes referred to as autoecholalia) and echolalia. Jargon or unintelligible speech may be noted, and there may be sudden shouting or low mumbling. Eventually syntax and phonology become incorrect and only jargon remains (Bayles & Boone, 1979).

As the client's language deteriorates, the need for communication becomes greater. The greatest challenge in working with the Alzheimer's client is helping the client maintain contact with the outside world by devising new methods of communication.

A Functional Communication Program for Managing the Alzheimer's Client

When outlining a course of action for anyone with a disease such as Alzheimer's, it is always wise to remember that all parties involved have needs that must be met and attitudes that may not always forward those needs. Much has been written about the need for intervention in cases of dementia (Mace & Rabins, 1981; Rabins, 1984; Wasow, 1986). In general the focus has been on family needs and family support, with little attention to therapy procedures suitable for the individual who has the disease.

In the past, the attitude toward treating the Alzheimer's client has been one of negativism and inevitable failure. "Why try to teach someone who can't learn?" and "You can't stay ahead of the disease" are among the common expressions of this attitude. Its effect has been to shift the focus of need for therapy away from the demented client and to create a new category of client, the family member who is caught in a never-ending spiral of increasing helplessness. Those interventions that did focus on the demented individual were aimed at alleviating behavioral problems. Families were left to their own devices in designing strategies that might ease some of the functional problems of the Alzheimer's client.

Despite this prevalence of negativism, data (Corkin et al., 1981; McEvoy & Patterson, 1986; Davis, 1986) show that, contrary to earlier beliefs, Alzheimer's clients can and do learn. This evidence highlights the need for the professional to redirect the focus of therapy back to the Alzheimer's client.

Cognitive training has been used with cognitively impaired persons with some success (Dunkle, 1984). Language analysis also has been used in planning and management strategies (Schwartz et al., 1979). Bayles & Boone (1982) suggested that strategies such as memory aids and shorter, less complex sentences can possibly improve functioning. Bartol (1979) emphasized the importance of nonverbal communication in dealing with Alzheimer's patients and compiled a list of guidelines for nurse–patient communication. There is little doubt as to the importance of and the need for working with the Alzheimer's person to improve communication and function.

In recognition of the need for an innovative program in communication suitable for use with Alzheimer's clients, a strategy has been designed that is based on the client's functional needs. Since a major obstacle in working with the Alzheimer's client is the need for frequent reinforcement, the client's caregiver is included as an equal partner in the therapy process. Thus the major focus of the therapy program is on both the individual that has the disease and the caregiver. The caregiver here is defined as any significant other having close, frequent contact with the demented individual who is willing to accept the role. When working in an outpatient setting, the caregiver must be present at all therapy sessions. In the long-term care setting, the caregiver is generally the certified nursing assistant (CNA). It is not always possible, however, to have the CNA present for the entire session. In such cases, the clinician must allow sufficient time to train the CNA in the appropriate techniques either at the end of each session or during an appropriate activity.

The lesson plans included in Unit 8 were developed in response to the need of professionals seeking therapy techniques suitable for dementia clients living in the community. To succeed, the lessons require the cooperation not only of the Alzheimer's client but of the family member or other caregiver and the professional who will teach the lesson. The therapy program presented here represents a departure from traditional programs in several aspects. Unlike the lessons given in most traditional communications programs, these lessons are based on the client's ADL needs. They make use of real objects in real situations. Further, the program requires the presence of a third party. Although it is possible to teach some of the lessons, such as the writing lesson, in a clinical setting, a more natural setting is recommended. The lessons in Unit 8 are well-suited for use in home care and for higher level residents of assisted living facilities.

In determining whether or not professionals and family members will accept the concept of sharing the burden of therapy, a survey of professionals and family members was conducted (Glickstein & Raiff, 1985). Both groups were asked whether family members should be part of the therapy process of the Alzheimer's client as evaluators or as part of an ongoing treatment plan. Professionals were asked whether they ever involved family members in the therapy process of the Alzheimer's client. Both professionals and family members agreed that they should work together and that families should be involved in the therapy process, but most professionals said that they never discussed test results with family members and would not involve them directly in therapy. The reasons offered ranged from "family members have enough to do" to "they wouldn't understand what I am doing." Many professionals were clearly uncomfortable with the idea of having a family member share the responsibilities of evaluation and treatment that they viewed as theirs.

A small number of family members agreed with the assessment of most of the professionals that the caregivers have enough to do. The majority of family members, however, believed that including them in the therapy process would be a positive step in helping both the family and the demented client. Many family members expressed resentment at receiving what they considered inadequate feedback. Consequently, those family members who have played an active role in the therapy process have reported positive feelings regarding treatment procedures.

Although improvement in functional communication skills for ADLs can help the Alzheimer's client and the family members improve their quality of life, it does not negate the fact that eventually the disease will progress to the point where the individual will no longer be able to function. Neither does it diminish the great need for ongoing family support. Integrating family members into the therapy process is a logical step in helping the family, and especially the caregiver, to function better while focusing on the therapy needs of the Alzheimer's client.

There are occasions when someone other than the family member will be designated as the primary caregiver. For example, Alzheimer's clients residing in a nursing home will have more frequent contact with aides and nursing staff than with family members. While the lesson plans presented in Unit 8 may suit some long-term care residents, it is more likely that the Action Oriented Program for Persons with Cognitive Disabilities (AOPPCD) presented in Unit 9 would be better suited to the majority of these clients. This does not negate the family's need for information or to share in what is happening. Regardless of the setting, when the family member does not have primary responsibility for the client's ADL needs, a third party would be designated the caregiver during therapy sessions.

Functional Assessment of Activities of Daily Living and Communication Skills

To design a program of therapy that would provide the greatest benefit to both the Alzheimer's client and the caregiver, it is necessary to evaluate not only communication skills but the client's ability to function independently; these areas could reflect the greatest gain from therapeutic intervention and training in the functional skills needed most to improve the client's and caregiver's quality of life. The therapist should complete this evaluation before instituting any plan of therapy by means of an instrument that will measure functional ability and disability.

"Functional impairment is the decreased ability to meet one's own needs, including the functions allowing mobility, cognition, eating, toileting, dressing, hygiene, shopping, cooking and managing money" (Besdine, 1983, p. 651). Functional impairment is a primary sign in the diagnosis of dementia. Assessment of the client's functional status must take into consideration premorbid as well as current abilities. Many disciplines, including occupational therapy, physical therapy, nursing, and social work, have contributed to the development of instruments to measure functional status in various settings. The information gathered through these measures is needed as part of the overall evaluation to help determine a course of action for the client. In choosing a particular instrument, the therapist should decide on the type and purpose of the information being sought as well as the rapidity and ease of administration of the instrument.

UNIDIMENSIONAL MEASURES OF FUNCTIONAL ABILITY

The first attempt to classify the functional capacity of the elderly was accomplished by the Research Bureau of the Welfare Council of New York City in 1934 (Krauss, 1962). The scale employed a four-fold classification of disability ranging from "no obvious disability" to "patient bedridden or confined to a chair." The reliability of this type of scale was shown to be low (Hutchinson et al., 1979). The first major breakthrough in the measurement of functional ability of adults came with the development of the IADL scale (Katz et al., 1963). Currently, there are multiple tools in use and under investigation for usefulness, reliability, and validity.

Index of Activities of Daily Living Scale

The development of the IADL scale was a significant departure from early undifferentiated scales (Katz et al., 1963). The scale was one of the first to define impairment categories and to establish its reliability. It consists of ratings of independence or dependence in six functions: feeding, continence, transfer skills, toileting, dressing, and bathing. Each area is rated 0 to 2 (no assistance to maximum assistance), and overall performance is summarized as grades A through G, where A is the most independent and G the most dependent grade. As originally conceived, the IADL scale requires a skilled observer to rate the client's performance on the basis of personal observations and a series of questions.

The purpose of the observations is to determine the degree of assistance the client received or whether the client functioned alone; assistance is defined as active personal assistance, directive assistance, or supervision. In considering the evaluation the actual existence of assistance is considered, and no evaluation or comments are made as to the potential of the client to function more independently, thereby disallowing differentiation between a client who is unable to perform a task and one who has an overly protective caregiver.

Physical Self-Maintenance Scale

The Physical Self-Maintenance Scale (PSMS) developed by Lawton and Brody (1969) includes the additional items of ambulation and grooming not found on the IADL scale. It further differs from the IADL scale in that it is designed to be administered by any health professional by means of various informants as opposed to direct observation, making it more flexible than the IADL scale. The PSMS offers the additional advantage of a single assessment that is appropriate for use in different settings.

Barthel Index

The Barthel Index (BI), as originally conceived, is a tool for evaluation of personal self care of patients prior to admission to, and discharge from, a rehabilitation hospital (Mahoney & Barthel, 1965). It is a measure of disability rather than ability. The index is a ten-item scale that includes feeding, transfer skills, toileting, bathing, ambulation, dressing, use of stairs, personal hygiene, and continence of bowel and bladder. The values assigned to each item are based on the time and amount of actual physical assistance required if the individual is unable to perform the activity. Each item on the ten-item scale is rated independently and the combined total is the index measure of independence in personal self-care. The lower the overall score, the greater the assistance needed. Thus a score of 0 would indicate someone who is incontinent, must be fed, dressed, bathed, and so on. A score of 100 indicates no assistance needed in self-care. The BI makes no assessment regarding the individual's ability to live alone or function in the community.

Modified Barthel Index

The Barthel Index as modified by Granger and colleagues (1979) measures the degree of independence in performing activities of daily living as well as independence in self-care. Each item is scored independently and a combined score of overall function is achieved. Combined scores range from 0 to 100. The higher the score the more independently the person can function. Fortinsky and coworkers (1981) found that the individual task scores on the modified Barthel Index have the ability to identify personal care needs and to pinpoint the need for support to perform specific tasks necessary for ADL in the home, such as light housecleaning.

MULTIDIMENSIONAL MEASURES

More recent developments in functional assessment have been the use of scales for understanding the needs of the individual for long-term care in the home setting. These comprehensive test batteries are designed to evaluate most or all of the areas of medical problems, functional disabilities, psychological status, and social network and needs.

Grauer and Birnbom (1975) constructed a multidimensional functional rating scale that includes positive items to assess the individual's ability to function and the support offered by personal contacts and public facilities. Among the most widely known programs to have developed such test batteries are the Older Americans Resources and Services questionnaire (OARS) and the Comprehensive Assessment and Referral Evaluation (CARE). The addition of social parameters to these tests adds a dimension not found in other scales.

Older Americans Resources and Services

The OARS multidimensional functional assessment questionnaire (Fillenbaum & Smyer, 1981) was the first publicized attempt to assess sensitively overall functioning and service utilization in a manner suitable for both current assessment and predictive purposes (Comptroller General of the United States, 1979). Developed initially in response to a request by the President's Commission on Aging to examine alternatives to institutionalization (Maddox, 1972), the OARS questionnaire permits both an overall assessment of personal functioning and an assessment of service utilization. Part A is designed to assess overall personal functioning on each of five dimensions: social, economic, mental health, physical health, and self-care capacity. The questionnaire is administered by a trained professional and requires approximately 45 minutes. Because of the length of time needed to administer the questionnaire and the complexity of its construction, the OARS is seldom used in its entirety.

Functional Assessment Inventory

The Functional Assessment Inventory (FAI) is an abbreviated modification of the OARS questionnaire. The FAI contains 11 distinct sections and offers several advantages for use with Alzheimer's clients over the OARS questionnaire. The first part of the inventory is the SPMSQ, which is used to determine whether the subject can reliably complete the remainder of the test or whether an informant will have to be used (Pfeiffer, 1975). The SPMSQ is administered by a trained interviewer through a face-to-face interview.

The FAI contains ten fewer items than the OARS questionnaire. Other changes include fewer response categories for selected items, a modified coding scheme, and two semantic differential rating scales measuring life satisfaction and self-esteem (Cairl et al., 1983).

Comprehensive Assessment and Referral Evaluation

According to its originators (Gurland et al., 1978), the CARE is a semistructured interview guide and inventory of defined ratings. The dimensions covered are somewhat different from the OARS questionnaire and the FAI in that nutritional status is considered as a separate dimension. The interview consists of a series of printed questions that the interviewer reads aloud to the interviewee. The questions fall into five categories: psychiatric, medical, nutritional, economic, and social. Evaluation time is approximately $1\frac{1}{2}$ hours. This is considerably longer than the time needed for the OARS questionnaire or the FAI, making the CARE impractical for routine use.

Hebrew Rehabilitation Center for Aged (HRCA) Vulnerability Index

The HRCA Vulnerability Index was developed from a sample of elderly tenants living alone in public housing developments. It was derived from interdisciplinary clinical team judgments of functional status but is now based on self-reported (or proxy) information (Morris et al., 1984). It is intended to be a rapid and easily applied method of identifying high-need elderly persons within the community.

The index is based on a system for scoring the responses to ten questions asked of the person being screened. The final score is used as a substitute for clinical judgment concerning physical functioning impairment status. The major features of this scale are the addition of the environmental aspect and the simple scoring system.

Structural Assessment of Independent Living Skills

The Structural Assessment of Independent Living Skills (SAILS) is a task performance test developed to measure the independent living skills of persons with dementia (see Exhibit 6–1). The test consists of 50 tasks divided into 10 groups of 5 items each. Items measured include dressing, motor skills, social interaction, and cognition. Administration time is approximately one hour but may take longer. Scoring is done as the test is administered. Each task is scored on the basis of accuracy and time needed for completion. There is a 4-point rating scale with 0 representing the lowest score and 3 the highest. Each section receives a total and all of the subtotals are combined to give a grand total (overall) score. The scores range from a high of 150 (no impairment) downward. The lower the score, the greater the impairment.

Summary

Ideally, functional assessment should be part of an ongoing continuum of care that includes uniform measures of function. Current measures of function vary from setting to setting and service to service, however, causing the outcome evaluation to be dependent on the data source (Rubenstein et al., 1984), the service, and the method of data collection.

Current measures of functional assessment generally include items concerning the individual's capability for self-care in increasing degrees of independence or dependence; the items range from basic ADLs such as feeding and toileting to the ability to travel and shop for groceries independently. The functional assessment of the abilities to carry out ADLs plays an important part in determining the course of action to be taken with the Alzheimer's client.

The need for assessment goes beyond the ability to use a washcloth and soap, because as Davis (1986) has said, "The world is full of potential hazards for Alzheimer's victims" (p. 20). Is the client able to identify hot and cold water taps? Furthermore, can the client use a knife without being harmed? Are there visual perceptual problems that might make using the stairs hazardous? Is the client capable of leaving the home environment alone? These are all questions that an in-depth functional assessment

Exhibit 6–1 Structural Assessment of Independent Living Skills (SAILS)

Scoring Form

Name: _____ Date: _____

Age: _____ Sex: _____ Handedness: _____ Education: _____ Examiner: _____

Diagnosis: _____

Note: If patient is unable to complete task, assign maximum time of 60″ unless otherwise indicated.

Motor Tasks

Fine Motor Skills | Time: | Score:

Task	Time:	Score:
1. Picks up coin 0 = drops two; 1 = drops one; 2 = slow; 3 = normal (8″)		
2. Removes wrappers 0 = needs assistance; 1 = tears one or more; 2 = slow; 3 = normal (35″)		
3. Cuts with scissors 0 = can't cut; 1 = off line; 2 = slow; 3 = normal (32″)		
4. Folds letter and places in envelope 0 = can't fold; 1 = doesn't fit; 2 = slow; 3 = normal (16″)		
5. Uses key in lock 0 = can't insert; 1 = can't unlock; 2 = slow; 3 = normal (13″)		

Subtotal:

Gross Motor Skills | Time: | Score:

Task	Time:	Score:
1. Stands up from sitting 0 = unable; 1 = uses arms of chair; 2 = slow; 3 = normal (2″)		
2. Opens and walks through door 0 = unable; 1 = needs door held open; 2 = slow; 3 = normal (5″)		
3. Regular gait 0 = unable; 1 = assistive device; 2 = slow; 3 = normal (6″) Time 1) ___ 2) ___ Mean ___ Steps 1) ___ 2) ___ Mean ___		
4. Tandem gait 0 = unable, steps off 4 or more times; 1 = steps off 2–3 times; 2 = slow (1step off allowed); 3 = normal (9″) Time 1) ___ 2) ___ Mean ___ Steps off line 1) ___ 2) ___ Mean ___		
5. Transfers object across room 0 = drops; 1 = inaccurate placement; 2 = slow; 3 = normal (6″) Time 1) ___ 2) ___ Mean ___		

Subtotal:

continues

Exhibit 6–1 continued

Dressing Skills   Time: Score:

1. Puts on shirt (maximum = 120″) 0 = can't put on or button; 1 = misaligned; 2 = slow; 3 = normal (86″)	
2. Buttons cuffs of shirt 0 = unable; 1 = one cuff; 2 = slow; 3 = normal (45″)	
3. Puts on jacket 0 = can't put it on; 1 = needs help with zipper; 2 = slow; 3 = normal (27″)	
4. Ties shoelaces 0 = unable/wrong feet; 1 = knot comes undone; 2 = slow; 3 = normal (9″)	
5. Puts on gloves 0 = unable; 1 = one hand; 2 = slow; 3 = normal (21″)	

Subtotal:

Eating Skills   Time: Score:

1. Drinks from glass 0 = unable; 1 = spills; 2 = slow; 3 = normal (3″)	
2. Transfers food with spoon 0 = unable; 1 = drops; 2 = slow; 3 = normal (11″)	
3. Cuts with fork and knife 0 = unable; 1 = drops; 2 = slow; 3 = normal (16″)	
4. Transfer food with fork 0 = unable; 1 = drops; 2 = slow; 3 = normal (16″)	
5. Transfers liquid with spoon 0 = unable; 1 = spills; 2 = slow; 3 = normal (13″)	

Subtotal:

Total Motor Time _____   Total Motor Score _____

Cognitive Tasks

Expressive Language   Score:

1. Quality of expression 0 = severe < 25%; 1 = moderate 25%–90%; 3 = intact	
2. Repetition 0 = no items; 1 = 1 item; 2 = 2 items; 3 = all 3 items	
3. Object naming 0 = 3 or less; 1 = 4 items; 2 = 5 items; 3 = all 6 items	
4. Writes legible note 0 = illegible; 1 = 1 item; 2 = 2 items; 3 = all 3 items	
5. Completes application form 0 = 3 or less; 1 = 4 items; 2 = 5 items; 3 = all 6 items	

Subtotal:

Receptive Language   Score:

1. Reads and follows printed instructions 0 = none; 1 = 1 item; 2 = 2 items; 3 = all 3 items	
2. Understands written material 0 = none; 1 = 1–4 items; 2 = 5 items; 3 = 6 items Article 1: Correct 1) ___ 2) ___ 3) ___ Article 2: Correct 1) ___ 2) ___ 3) ___	

continues

Exhibit 6–1 continued

3. Understands common signs 0 = none; 1 = 1 item; 2 = 2 items; 3 = 3 items	
4. Follows verbal directions 0 = none; 1 = 1 item; 2 = 2 items; 3 = 3 items 1) Touch shoulder; 2) Hands on table, close eyes; 3) Draw circle, hand pencil, fold paper	
5. Identifies named objects 0 = none; 1 = 1 item; 2 = 2 items; 3 = all 3 items	

Subtotal:

Time and Orientation   Score:

1. States time on clock (6:14) 0 = off over 1 hour; 1 = off within 1 hour; 2 = off 10 minutes; 3 = correct within 1 minute	
2. Calculates time interval (until 7:30) 0 = off 1 hour; 1 = off within 1 hour; 2 = off within 15 minutes; 3 = correct within 1 minute	
3. States time of alarm setting (8:15) 0 = off 1 hour; 1 = off within 1 hour; 2 = off within 15 minutes; 3 = correct within 1 minute	
4. Locates current date on calendar 0 = incorrect month; 1 = correct month; 2 = correct week; 3 = correct date	
5. Correctly reads calendar 0 = none; 1 = 1 item; 2 = 2 items; 3 = all 3 items 1) Fridays; 2) Day of 15th; 3) 2nd Monday	

Subtotal:

Money-Related Skills   Score:

1. Counts money 0 = none; 1 = 1 item; 2 = 2 items; 3 = all 3 items 1) 35 cents; 2) 95 cents; 3) $1.41	
2. Makes change 0 = none; 1 = 1 item; 2 = 2 items; 3 = all 3 items 1) ($.75 from $1.00) = $.25 ___; 2) ($.41 from $.50) = $.09 ___; 3) ($2.79 from $5.00) = $2.21	
3. Understands monthly utility bill 0 = none; 1 = 1 item; 2 = 2 items; 3 = all 3 items 1) (Light Co.) ___; 2) ($38.46) ___; 3) (3/6/87) ___	
4. Writes check 0 = 2 or less; 1 = 1–3 items; 2 = 4 items; 3 = all 5 items 1) Date; 2) Payee; 3) Numerical amount; 4)Written amount; 5) Signature	
5. Understands checkbook 0 = none; 1 = 1 item; 2 = 2 items; 3 = all 3 items 1) Checks on August 11; 2) Check #355; 3) Balance ($440.00)	

Subtotal:

Total Cognitive Score _____

Instrumental Activities   Score:

1. Uses telephone book 0 = none; 1 = 1 item; 2 = 2 items; 3 = all 3 items	
2. Dials telephone number 0 = cannot handle phone; 1 = misdials number; 2 = needs help to read; 3 = correctly reads and dials	

continues

Exhibit 6–1 continued

3. Understands medication label 0 = none; 1 = 1 item; 2 = 2 items; 3 = all 3 items	
4. Opens medication container 0 = can't open two; 1 = can't open one; 2 = needs cue; 3 = normal	
5. Follows simple recipe 0 = unable; 1 = 1 step; 2 = 2 steps; 3 = all 3 steps	

Subtotal: _____

Social Interaction   Score:

1. Responds to greeting and farewell 0 = none; 1 = 1 item; 2 = 2 items; 3 = all 3 items	
2. Responds to request for information 0 = none; 1 = 1 item; 2 = 2 items; 3 = all 3 items	
3. Responds to social directives 0 = none; 1 = 1 item; 2 = 2 items; 3 = all 3 items	
4. Requests needed information 0 = none; 1 = 1 item; 2 = 2 items; 3 = all 3 items	
5. Understands nonverbal expression 0 = none; 1 = 1item; 2 = 2 items; 3 = all 3 items	

Subtotal: _____

Grand Total Score _____

Source: Reprinted with permission from R.K. Mahurin, B.H. DeBettings, and F.J. Pirozzolo, Structured Assessment of Independent Living Skills: Preliminary Report of a Performance Measure of Functional Abilities in Dementia, *Journal of Gerontology,* Vol. 46, No. 2, pp. 58–66, © 1991, the Gerontological Society of America.

should address if safety and well-being are the major focus. In addition to dementia, the client may have sensory deficits, such as auditory or visual loss, that must be considered when evaluating his or her current status and needs.

Family reports and rater observations of behavior are the most frequent methods of determining functional assessment, but information learned from such assessments may vary considerably according to the informant (Rubenstein et al., 1984). As the demand for treatment increases, objective measures such as the Barthel Index (Fortinsky et al., 1981) are becoming more important in evaluating and documenting client needs and changes in functional status over time. The use of these measures should become equally important in planning and evaluating therapy.

IDENTIFYING THE FUNCTIONAL COMMUNICATION LEVEL OF THE DEMENTIA CLIENT

Diagnosis and treatment of Alzheimer's disease is a team effort, yet the assessment of communication skills in dementia clients has been an area frequently overlooked by speech pathologists, despite the fact that these skills are affected early and grow progressively worse over the course of the disease. A speech-language pathologist, like other individual members of the diagnostic team, does not diagnose Alzheimer's disease. It is the speech-language pathologist's job to evaluate and to determine whether there is a communication loss and the nature of this loss, to make recommendations regarding speech and language prognosis, and to decide whether therapy could be of benefit. The results of the evaluation are then used by the primary physician or, preferably, the multidisciplinary team in making the overall diagnosis and planning a course of action.

When assessing a client with a suspected dementia, the therapist needs to consider the nature of the disease in order to select appropriate test materials. The tools chosen should include at least one measure of functional communication. Exhibit 6–2 is a comparison of the communication and related components of some well-known functional assessment measures.

Because Alzheimer's clients do not show the classic patterns of aphasia, test selection can be problematic for the speech-language pathologist. Tests that allow the client sufficient time and opportunity to display areas of competence as well as areas of loss are needed. It is important to sample the individual's auditory comprehension, narrative writing (e.g., writing a paragraph describing a picture), and writing from dictation (e.g., writing sentences from dictation) along with speech output, as these areas are affected early in the course of the disease. Testing time is also a factor since most dementia clients cannot attend for a long enough period to complete a standard battery of tests. With these factors in mind, the clinician might wish to consider some or all of the following test battery for use with dementia clients: (1) the Boston Diagnostic Aphasia Examination (BDAE; Goodglass & Kaplan, 1972), (2) the Fuld Object-Memory Evaluation and the Fuld adaptation of the mental status test of Blessed and associates (Fuld, 1983), and (3) the Functional Communication Profile (FCP) (Sarno, 1969). Other tests yielding similar information are available, and the reader should not feel constrained to use any single test or test battery. The tests listed here have been used successfully with dementia clients.

Boston Diagnostic Aphasia Examination

The BDAE has become one of the most familiar tests among speech-language pathologists. The length of time needed to complete the test, more than 90 minutes if supplementary tests are given, makes it difficult to administer at a single meeting, however. At the initial session the therapist should select sections from the BDAE to use with the client that yield information regarding language and speech comprehension such as naming, repetition tasks, responses to yes or no questions, and so on. On the basis of the results of these selected tests, the therapist then selects specific areas, such as reading, writing, or number concepts, for more in-depth evaluation, possibly at a later date.

Fuld Object-Memory Evaluation and Fuld Adaptation of Blessed's Mental Status Test

Fuld (1983) suggested that, in the early and middle stages of Alzheimer's disease, inappropriate recurrences of a response to earlier test items is an indication of Alzheimer's disease. For example, the client may intrude names of people into the attempted recall of a list of objects named earlier. The now-inappropriate words are called word intrusions. This term is used to make the distinction between incorrect responses that have occurred earlier and those that have not. Minimum test procedures acceptable when eliciting word intrusions are the object-naming section, one or two recall trials, and the rapid categorized word-listing part of the Fuld Object-Memory Evaluation, along with the mental status examination (Fuld, 1983).

Word intrusions are most likely to occur on the Fuld Object-Memory Evaluation (Fuld, 1983). An increase of more than four error points on the Fuld adaptation of Blessed's mental status test is significant. Clients with Alzheimer's disease most often make errors on the date, month, year, and day (temporal portion) but can correctly state their own birth date. The most common type of intrusion is the recall of the client's own birth date when asked for today's date.

Exhibit 6–2 Communication and Related Components of Sample Functional Assessment Measures

Measure (reference)	NONE	Receptive/expressive communication dichotomy	Hearing sensitivity	Central auditory processing	Auditory comprehension	Speech production (e.g., intelligibility)	Language production	Nonverbal communication (e.g., gestures, augmentative)	Reading	Writing	Voice	Fluency	Cognitive processes	Swallowing (may be addressed in "feeding" category)
ADL and Multidimensional Measures:														
Index of ADL (Katz et al, 1963).	+													
Barthel Index (Mahoney & Barthel, 1965).	+													
Patient Appraisal and Care Evaluation-2nd version (PACE-II): Impairments Section (U.S. DHEW, 1978).		+	+											
Older American Research and Service Center Instrument (OARS): ADL (Duke University, 1978).	+													
Functional Health Status of the Institutionalized Elderly: ADL (Mossey & Tisdale. 1979).	+													
Rehabilitation Measures:														
Functional Independence Measure (FIM) (Hamilton et al., 1987).		+[a]											+	+
Good Samaritan Rehabilitation Center's Program Evaluation Functional Assessment Scale (Snope, 1973).			+	+	+	+[b]	+[c]	+				+	+	
Revised Level of Rehabilitation Scale (LORS-II) (Carey & Posavac, 1982).					+	+	+	+	+	+			+	+
Patient Evaluation and Conference System (PECS) (Harvey & Jellinek, 1979, 1981).				+	+	+	+	+	+	+			+	+
New Medico Comprehensive Assessment Inventory for Rehabilitation (NM-CAIR) (Haffey & Johnston, 1988).				+	+	+	+	+	+	+			+	+
Speech-Language Pathology & Audiology Measures:														
Functional Communication Profile (FCP) (Sarno, 1969).				+	+		+	+	+	+			+	
Communicative Abilities in Daily Living (CADL) (Holland, 1980).[d]				+	+		+	+	+	+			+	
ASHA's Program Evaluation System (PES): Functional Communication Measures (Larkins, 1987).		+		+	+	+	+	+	+	+	+	+	+	+

(a) Considers auditory, visual comprehension, and verbal nonverbal expression in ratings
(b) Includes a separate assessment of "pragmatics"
(c) Includes writing
(d) CADL is not communication modality-specific but taps above functions as indicated

Approximately 15 to 20 minutes are needed to complete the evaluation. When word intrusions are not observed or when they are either profuse or self-corrected, diseases other than Alzheimer's should be suspected.

Functional Communication Profile

Of paramount importance in the day-to-day life of the dementia client is function. There are few objective measures of communication performance that detail functional ability. The FCP is a practical, easy-to-administer test aimed at determining functional communication abilities in daily living situations. It was designed in 1956 as part of a battery of tests used to evaluate brain-damaged adults. The profile has 45 items related to communication behaviors, which are considered common functions of everyday life. A nine-point scale is used to rate each behavior on the basis of the therapist's informal interaction with the client in a conversational situation. The therapist evaluates the client in five categories which are subdivided in order of their complexity. The categories are *movement* (ability to imitate movement, use of gestures); *speaking* (saying greetings, giving directions); *understanding* (awareness of speech, understanding simple conversation with one person); *reading* (reading comprehension—ability to read single words and magazine articles—but not the ability to read out loud); and *other* (writing and copying, time orientation, handling money, and calculation ability).

The primary purpose of the FCP is to obtain a quantitative measure of functional communication regardless of the client's degree of impairment. Although it has not been standardized for a dementia population, it is a useful tool in evaluating the functional communication of the client. By making use of objects in the environment, the test can be helpful when planning behavioral therapies.

Functional Communication Measure

The Functional Communication Measure (FCM) (Exhibit 6–3) is a data-collecting instrument being developed by the American Speech-Language-Hearing Association (ASHA) Task Force on Treatment

---

Exhibit 6–3 Functional Communication Measure

Speech Production Disorder

Level 0 Unable to test.

Level 1 Production of speech is unintelligible.

Level 2 Spontaneous production of speech is limited in intelligibility. Some automatic speech and imitative words or consonant/vowel (CV) combinations may be intelligible.

Level 3 Spontaneous production of speech consists primarily of automatic words or phrases with inconsistent intelligibility.

Level 4 Spontaneous production of speech is intelligible at the phrase level in familiar contexts; out of context, speech generally is unintelligible unless self-cueing and self-monitoring strategies are applied.

Level 5 Spontaneous production of speech is intelligible for meeting daily living needs; out of context, periodic repetition, rephrasing, or provision of a cue is required.

Level 6 Spontaneous production of speech is intelligible in and out of context, but the production is sometimes distorted.

Level 7 Production of speech is normal in all situations.

continues

Exhibit 6–3 continued

Voice Disorder

Level 0   Unable to test.

Level 1   Voice production (pitch, quality, loudness) is nonfunctional for communicating.

Level 2   Voice production is functional for brief episodes; most communication must be accomplished by nonvocal means.

Level 3   Voice production is unreliable, although some vocal communication may occur in limited contexts.

Level 4   Appropriate voice production is limited. Self-monitoring and self-correcting skills are inconsistent. Voice quality is distracting to most listeners.

Level 5   Appropriate voice production (pitch, quality, loudness) is consistent in most contexts. Self-correcting skills are used appropriately. Voice quality is distracting to some listeners.

Level 6   Voice production is appropriate in most situations, although minimal difficulty may occur.

Level 7   Voice production is normal for all speaking situations.

Disorder of Rate, Rhythm, or Fluency

Level 0   Unable to test.

Level 1   Speech rate, rhythm, or fluency makes speaking nonfunctional for speaker; listener cannot comprehend message.

Level 2   Speech rate, rhythm, or fluency is functional only for automatic words and phrases; listener's comprehension is severely limited and may be compounded by the speaker's facial grimaces, eye blinks, extraneous noises, etc.

Level 3   Speech rate, rhythm, or fluency interferes with comprehension of message at most times and in most environments; struggle, avoidance, and other coping behaviors may be observed.

Level 4   Speech rate, rhythm, or fluency impede listener's comprehension on a regular basis; struggle, avoidance, and other coping behaviors often accompany speaking efforts.

Level 5   Speech rate, rhythm, or fluency is appropriate at some times or in some environments; speaker is aware and frustrated; listener is distracted and may experience some difficulty in comprehending message.

Level 6   Speech rate, rhythm, or fluency is appropriate in most situations, although minimal difficulty may occur; self-monitoring/self-correction may be present; speaker is only mildly concerned or unaware of interruptions to the flow of speech; listener is mildly distracted, but comprehends message.

Level 7   Speech rate, rhythm, or fluency is normal in all situations.

Ability to Swallow Function

Level 0   Unable to test.

Level 1   Swallowing is not functional.

Level 2   Swallowing disorder prevents eating for all nutritional needs, but some swallowing is possible.

Level 3   Swallowing disorder prevents eating for a portion of nutritional needs and one-to-one supervision is required for eating.

Level 4   Swallowing disorder does not prevent eating to meet nutritional needs, although general supervision is required to ensure use of compensatory techniques.

Level 5   Swallowing is functional to meet nutritional needs, although self-monitoring and compensatory techniques are used.

Level 6   Swallowing is functional for most eating activity, although mild difficulty may occur periodically; additional time may be necessary for eating.

Level 7   Swallowing is normal in all situations.

Comprehension of Spoken Language

Level 0   Unable to test.

Level 1   No comprehension of spoken language.

continues

Exhibit 6–3 continued

Level 2   Comprehension of spoken language is limited to familiar words and/or phrases related to personal needs, although most responses are inaccurate or inappropriate.

Level 3   Comprehension of spoken language consists primarily of simple statements about personal topics, although repetition and/or rephrasing are required. Accuracy of comprehension is erratic.

Level 4   Comprehension of spoken language is limited to the primary activities of daily living needs and simple ideas and frequently requires repetition and/or rephrasing.

Level 5   Comprehension of spoken language is normal for activities of daily living, but limited in complexity of form, content, or use; self-monitoring is inconsistent.

Level 6   Comprehension of spoken language is normal in most situations, although minimal difficulty may occur; self-monitoring and self-correcting are present.

Level 7   Comprehension of spoken language is normal in all situations.

Production of Spoken Language

Level 0   Unable to test.

Level 1   No meaningful spoken language.

Level 2   Spoken language is limited to automatic and/or imitative words and phrases, although most attempts are inaccurate or inappropriate.

Level 3   Spoken language consists primarily of automatic speech with inconsistent words or phrases, although production may be accurate in imitation.

Level 4   Spoken language is limited to the communication of primary activities of daily living needs and simple ideas.

Level 5   Spoken language is functional for activities of daily living, but limited in complexity of form, content, or use; self-monitoring is inconsistent.

Level 6   Spoken language is functional in most situations, although minimal difficulty

may occur (e.g., word recall, latency of responding); self-monitoring and self-correcting are present.

Level 7   Spoken language is normal in all situations.

Comprehension of Written Language

Level 0   Unable to test.

Level 1   No comprehension of written language.

Level 2   Comprehension of written language is limited to familiar words and/or phrases related to personal needs, although most responses are inaccurate.

Level 3   Comprehension of written language consists primarily of words about personal topics, although cueing is required. Accuracy of comprehension is erratic.

Level 4   Comprehension of written language is limited to the primary activities of daily living needs and simple ideas; frequently requires cueing.

Level 5   Comprehension of written language is functional for activities of daily living, but limited in complexity of form, content, or use; self-monitoring is consistent.

Level 6   Comprehension of written language is functional in most situations; minimal difficulty may occur; self-monitoring and self-correcting are present.

Level 7   Comprehension of written language is normal in all situations.

Production of Written Language

Level 0   Unable to test.

Level 1   No production of written language.

Level 2   Production of written language is limited to the copying of numbers, letters, and/or words, although most attempts are distorted; spontaneous productions are inaccurate and/or illegible.

Level 3   Spontaneous productions of written language consist primarily of over-learned and/or familiar words, although copying may be normal.

continues

Exhibit 6–3 continued

Level 4   Production of written language is limited to words for activities of daily living and simple ideas.

Level 5   Production of written language is functional for activities of daily living, but limited in complexity of form, content, or use; self-monitoring is consistent.

Level 6   Production of written language is functional in most situations, although minimal difficulty may occur; self-monitoring and self-correcting are present.

Level 7   Production of written language is normal for all situations.

Cognitive Communication

Level 0   Unable to test.

Level 1   No meaningful cognitive communication.

Level 2   Cognitive communication is limited to brief episodes of appropriateness with minimal cueing; client is unaware of deficits.

Level 3   Cognitive communication is functional only for selected activities with supervision. Client is aware of deficits with cueing.

Level 4   Cognitive communication is functional only in a structured environment; supervision and/or cueing is necessary for activities of daily living needs and simple ideas. Client is aware of deficit.

Level 5   Cognitive communication is functional for activities of daily living, but limited in complexity; self-monitoring and use of compensatory strategies are inconsistent.

Level 6   Cognitive communication is functional in most situations, although minimal difficulty may occur (e.g., complex problem solving, latency of response). Self-monitoring and self-correcting are present.

Level 7   Cognitive communication is normal in all situations.

Source: Reprinted with permission from ASHA Task Force on Treatment Outcomes and Cost Effectiveness, *Users Guide for Pilot Study Phase 1,* Unpublished document of the National Treatment Outcomes Data Collection Project of the American Speech-Language-Hearing Association, © 1995, ASHA.

Outcomes and Cost Effectiveness to measure functional outcomes. The scale consists of 13 areas of communication/swallowing. Each area is rated on a scale of 0 to 7. When used as part of an initial evaluation, the scale could offer a practical baseline evaluation of the individual's functional status.

Rating Scale of Communication in Cognitive Decline

According to Bollinger and Hardiman (1991), the Rating Scale of Communication in Cognitive Decline (RSCCD) was developed as an outgrowth of a clinical need. The rating scale includes a total of 20 items divided into Verbal and Nonverbal sections. Each item is rated on a five-point scale that designates the frequency of occurrence of a given communicative behavior. The RSCCD presumes an existing diagnosis of dementia. The items on the scale reflect cognitive-communicative behaviors rather than language per se. Behavioral ratings are based on *observed* and/or *reported* communication behaviors. Behaviors include expressing ideas, physical-emotional needs, writing messages, and staying on the topic when talking. The authors report that the RSCCD correlates highly with both the Mini-Mental Status and the Global Deterioration Scale. The scale is short, quick, and to the point.

Working with Dementia Clients Living in the Community

As soon as the evaluation for functional ADL and communication skills has been completed and the diagnosis determined, a treatment plan should be formulated. This unit introduces a series of specific lesson plans (contained in Unit 8) designed to be used with clients diagnosed as having probable Alzheimer's disease or other dementia and who are living in a community-based environment.

TWO CASE HISTORIES

Steve

Steve was 56 years old when he was diagnosed as having Alzheimer's disease. At the time of his diagnosis, he was working for a local steel company. He was married and had three children. The series of events leading up to his diagnosis were unusual and for a period of time made diagnosis more difficult.

After Steve's 21-year-old retarded son died unexpectedly, Steve and his wife closed their house and went on a vacation. Upon their return, they found that the house had burned to the ground. Shortly after that, Steve's mother-in-law died.

Forced to live with his daughter so that he would be close to work, Steve found himself unable to concentrate. His job performance dropped, and he became a hazard to himself and his coworkers. Steve's wife complained that he "couldn't keep his mind on what he was doing." Steve complained, "Things looked funny. I couldn't read."

A routine physical examination was inconclusive, and a diagnosis of depression was offered. Approximately six months later, Steve discovered that he was having trouble dressing. He was unable to tie his tie or his shoe laces. Upon his return to his physician, Steve was sent for a complete medical examination and psychological evaluation. At this time he was diagnosed with probable early Alzheimer's disease.

Exhibit 7–1 illustrates Steve's spontaneous writing in stage 1 of the disease. Note the repetition of the word "thank." In the first "thank" Steve substitutes the letter "t," which appears at the beginning of the word, for the letter "k." The slash through the letters "an" occurred when he tried to cross the final "t." The repetition of the word "thank" was not an attempt to start over. Note too, the intrusion of an extra letter in the words "you." At this time, placement of extra letters appeared to be a random occurrence. Steve, formerly a good speller, was unaware of his error on the word "evening." The content of the note is meaningful and there is good sentence structure. With the exception of his use of capitals to start a sentence, punctuation is lacking. The writing lesson (Lesson One) in Level I was developed to help Steve maintain contact with his son, who lived in another state.

Exhibit 7–2A illustrates Steve's spontaneous writing during stage 2 of the disease. In this stage, Steve was no longer able to write short sentences or to write to dictation. He was able to write the therapist's first name, Joan. When he was asked to write his name immediately after writing "Joan," however, the letters "oan" converged with the "Ste" of Steve. With successive trials and repetition of the directions, Steve could eventually write his name (Exhibit 7–2B).

The writing lesson (Lesson One) in Level II was designed to help Steve continue to use all of his resources in recalling people and events important to him. Exhibit 7–2B illustrates Steve's writing after a practice session.

Sara

The following example illustrates functional therapy in operation.

Sara, a 63-year-old retired bookkeeper, lived alone in a one-bedroom apartment located on the fifth floor of a small apartment building. Sara had never married. Her only living relative, a married sister,

---

Exhibit 7–1 Writing Sample of a Stage 1 Alzheimer's Client

Exhibit 7–2A   Writing Sample of a Stage 2 Alzheimer's Client without Practice

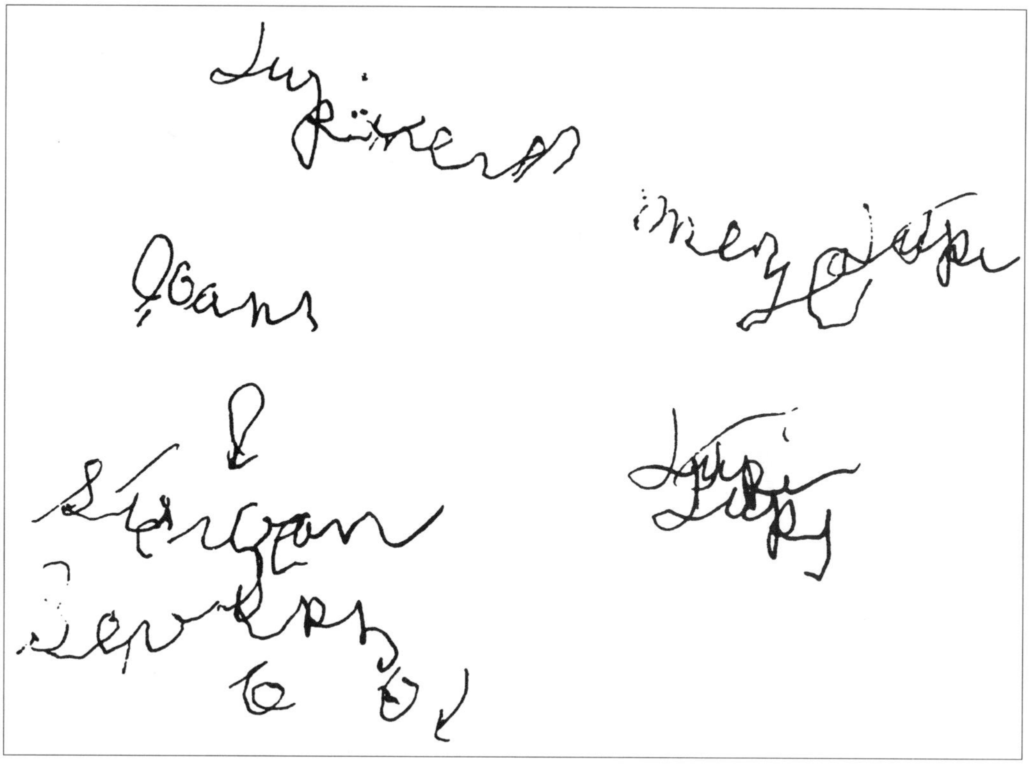

lived in a larger apartment on the same floor of the building. Sara had been thoroughly evaluated and diagnosed as being in the early stages of Alzheimer's disease. Sara's sister, Mary, was Sara's caregiver.

On several occasions, Sara had used the elevator in her building to go downstairs but was unable to find her way back to her apartment. She would get off on the wrong floor and try to enter other apartments. Sara was also having difficulty paying her bills, and she complained about her vision even though her ophthalmologist reported no organic visual dysfunction.

Evaluation of Sara's speech and language abilities indicated a generalized loss in language skills, particularly in basic arithmetic skills, ability to follow complex commands, and abstract thinking. Sara was able to identify colors, match numbers, and follow oral and written one-step instructions. On the functional evaluation Sara knew how to operate an elevator, and she had no difficulty pressing the correct number when asked to do so. She could not remember what floor to return to until she was told, however. In the course of conversation Sara mentioned that her favorite colors were lavender and yellow because they were "cheerful." She completed a brief note with the assistance of the therapist. In the note she said "I feel dum dum Help me."

Because Sara was motivated and still had sufficient ability to participate in a therapy program, the decision was made to work with both Sara (now designated the client) and her caregiver. After the information gained in both the formal and informal test modes was combined, the following therapy plan was carried out.

Exhibit 7–2B Writing Sample of a Stage 2 Alzheimer's Client with Practice

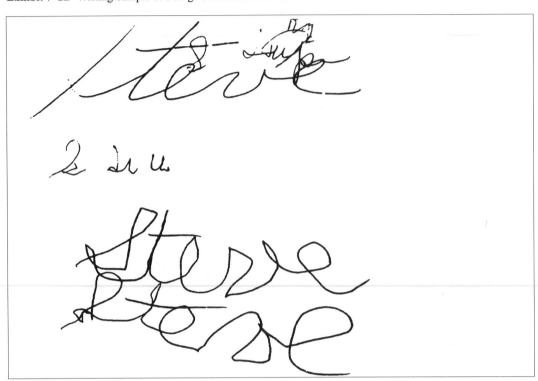

The client was assisted in using her residual skills to maintain her sense of independence. The client and her caregiver needed immediate help in two areas. The first was preventing the client from wandering out of her building and getting lost. The second was discovering an acceptable method for the client to write checks.

Since the apartment building in which the client and caregiver lived had a doorman, an obvious first step was to notify him of the client's condition and enlist his help in returning the client to her apartment or in notifying the caregiver, through the apartment intercom system, when he saw the client downstairs alone.

Since the client could identify numbers and colors, she was taught to place the number 1 on a yellow sticker and the number 5 on a lavender sticker. The therapist then helped the caregiver color-code the buttons on the building elevator to correspond to the colors used during the lessons. The next step was to have the client, caregiver, and therapist practice using the color-coded buttons on the elevator. (Eventually the yellow sticker was removed from the elevator panel, and only the lavender sticker remained.)

To help the client find her apartment once she got off the elevator, a large lavender sticker with the client's picture was posted on her apartment door. When the caregiver was satisfied that the client could find her way back to her apartment, the client was allowed to use the elevator alone. The doorman now assisted the client to the elevator, and she was allowed to return on her own.

The same color-coding technique was used to help the client in calling her caregiver on the telephone. Using a pink sticker on the "auto" button of a telephone with large numbers, the client practiced calling and talking to her caregiver.

To help the client and caregiver with check writing, facsimile checks were prepared. When the client was unable to write a check, the caregiver filled out the body of the check. The client, after reading the check aloud, signed it. The client then matched the name on the check to one in a ledger she kept and put a check mark next to that name. This procedure was important to the client because she had been a bookkeeper and insisted on "keeping books."

USING THE LESSON PLANS

The overall goals of the lesson plans are to improve the functional communication, defined simply as the ability to receive and use information in a purposeful manner, of the dementia client and to enhance the ability of the client to function successfully within a given environment. Each lesson is structured to focus on an event and its outcome rather than on particular communication skills. The lessons are suitable for use in both home care and institutional settings and need not be used exclusively by a speech-language pathologist. Other disciplines such as occupational therapy should find the techniques equally useful. To achieve success, it may be necessary to adapt the environment in an institutional setting. Exhibit 7–3 is a list of environmental considerations for treatment sessions.

The lessons take advantage of the mildly to moderately affected dementia client's ability to acquire and retain new information by introducing strategies that can be modified to suit his or her needs as the disease progresses. A word of caution: the clinician should not view these lessons as a linear progression from Lesson 1 to Lesson 6. Rather, the intent here is for the clinician to choose those items or concepts that are relevant to the client's current lifestyle and level of functioning and to design a meaningful program that will serve both client and caregiver in day-to-day activities.

Each lesson is designed around a specific activity based on the daily routine of the client. The lesson takes into account the current functional level of the client, the circumstances under which a particular task is to be performed, and the availability of a significant other (caregiver) to aid in task performance. The lessons are divided into four levels; the therapist will note that the same lesson is repeated in a modified format in different levels. The lessons all have the following general structural format that is carried throughout:

1. Identify the components/objects needed to achieve the stated goal. Some components and objects, such as personal grooming articles, can be used with clients throughout the course of the disease. Other objects, such as writing materials, are not suitable for later-stage clients. The degree of complexity in the lesson is not based on the number of objects used, but is based on the manner in which each object is treated.

Exhibit 7–3 Environmental Considerations for Treatment Sessions

• *Location of the area:*	Areas that have other activities or people passing through should be avoided.
• *Size of the area:*	A small work room or quiet work area is preferable.
• *Room contents:*	Rooms that are cluttered with unfamiliar objects can be distracting.
• *Noise level:*	Continual background noises act as a distraction to everyone.
• *Adequate lighting:*	Dim or flickering lights reduce concentration.
• *Availability:*	It is important to use the same room for every lesson. Changing rooms can cause confusion, which will reduce the lesson's effectiveness.

2. Associate the objects with symbolic representation, such as a picture or written material, in order to involve the client's visual and tactile skills as well as reading comprehension. In the earlier stages, the lesson for a daily routine utilizes real objects, such as a tooth brush, as well as pictures and printed representations. At each successive stage the object remains the same (toothbrush), but the representation is modified. By stage 3, only the actual object remains.
3. Encourage the client to motorically produce the word for the object—oral, written. At each stage the client is encouraged to demonstrate his or her ability to externalize information using a variety of modalities.
4. Identify the action associated with the object or verb. The complexity of the response requested from the client is determined by the client's functional ability. Thus a stage 1 client may be asked to describe, to write, and to demonstrate the action, while a stage 3 client may need some assistance in demonstrating.
5. Link the subject/object with the action. Linking affords the client an opportunity to make the connection between the materials used for instruction and the place it has in his or her own life. This is the critical final step in "training."
6. Reinforce this linkage by using the pictorial and written symbols in the actual ADL situation. Although a number of lessons in this unit are placed in a clinical setting, the client's home is equally suitable and in some instances may be preferred. In that case, linkage is made during the lesson and is an ongoing process.

Lessons introduced in Level I contain all the strategies used in the same lesson in Level II and Level III. By maintaining the stability of the routine, modifications that the client may need at a later stage are introduced early enough in the course of therapy for the client to acquire the new strategy. Thus, when the client is no longer functioning well enough to use the strategies outlined in Level I, he or she has already acquired the strategies needed for Level II. Of equal importance is the fact that the caregiver has acquired these same strategies and the methods to implement them. Therapists are encouraged to use the general format discussed above in formulating their own lessons for their clients. When using the lessons, all parties must understand both the nature of Alzheimer's disease and the intent of the lessons. The disease itself will not be modified. The goal is to help client and caregiver function better by making optimum use of current skills.

Each level begins with a description of the behaviors that are exhibited by an Alzheimer's client at that level. The levels used for the lesson plans are based on the four stages of Alzheimer's disease presented in Unit 2. The reader may refer to Unit 2 behavioral changes for a more detailed description of client behavior. The therapist is encouraged to pick and choose among the materials that best suit his or her purpose. If the client has difficulty with a lesson on the level chosen, the same lesson from a lower level should be tried. If the client is successful, the lesson should be repeated at the next session with one element from the next higher level introduced.

Under each lesson there are specific major objectives as well as general objectives listed. The general objectives are reinforced throughout the lessons and are identified under the *Comment* section of each lesson.

THE ROLE OF THE CAREGIVER

Even the mildly demented client has difficulty making the transition from task instruction to task performance. Therefore, to be effective, these lessons need reinforcement. To optimize reinforcement of the lessons, they must be used with the client and a caregiver under the direction of a trained professional (speech and language clinician or other health care professional) in any of the following settings: home care, rehabilitation center, day care, clinic, or nursing home. The caregiver is the individual who has the greatest amount of contact with the client and who is generally responsible for the client's well-being.

Most often spouses or close family members are the caregivers for clients living at home. For clients in institutional or residential settings, aides or volunteers other than family members are sometimes the primary caregivers. Thus the term as used in these lessons may be an aide at a long-term care facility responsible for grooming and feeding a particular patient, or a spouse needing instruction on how to maintain communication at home. Regardless of the setting, reinforcement is the caregiver's responsibility. Reinforcement means incorporating the lesson into the daily routine of both the client and caregiver. Because the lesson makes use of the current activities of the client and caregiver, reinforcement becomes part of a daily routine as opposed to time set aside for practice.

It is to the advantage of all involved that the caregiver be present during each therapy session so that the lesson can be repeated outside the training situation. The caregiver is not merely an observer; he or she must be an integral part of the lesson. To accomplish this, the caregiver must understand the goal of the lesson and how to reinforce the exercise.

IDENTIFYING THE FUNCTIONAL LEVEL OF THE DEMENTIA CLIENT

Just as there is currently no exact or certain method of diagnosing Alzheimer's disease, there is no exact or certain method of determining what stage an Alzheimer's client has reached. Before an appropriate plan of care can be outlined, however, the clinician must determine the client's current level of performance and have some reasonable expectations as to possible improvement. To aid the therapist in choosing appropriate lessons, each of the four levels begins with a section titled Functional Ability, which gives a description of behaviors that the therapist might observe and that would be helpful for him or her to know when planning activities. To succeed with a lesson on a given level, the client must, at a minimum, fit the description under Functional Ability for that level.

The inclusion of any behavior at any given level does not preclude that particular behavior from being present earlier or later in the course of the disease. The specific language behaviors listed are a composite of the language behaviors presented at two American Speech-Language-Hearing Association (ASHA) short courses on Alzheimer's disease, one by Cummings (1984b) and the second by Obler (1985). Additional behavioral descriptions were derived from Reisberg (1984), Schneck, Reisberg, and Ferris (1982), and material gathered from personal experience with families and dementia clients.

To determine which level is appropriate for the client, all outstanding features (positive and negative) of the evaluation data in the following areas should be listed: speech and language, cognitive tasks, orientation, number concept, memory, and ADLs. Any additional observations and information, such as concentration, particular interests, or routines, should also be listed. This list is then compared with the descriptions provided under "Functional Ability" at the beginning of each level of the lesson plan. Once the appropriate level for the client has been determined, the lesson that best suits the client's needs can then be chosen. As the disease progresses and the client's level of functional ability decreases, the lesson must be adapted to the changes with material drawn from the lessons in the next level.

Because of the highly variable nature of Alzheimer's disease, some clients' skills may overlap the various levels. If this is the case, the therapist must determine which items are suitable to the client's needs. At the beginning of Unit 7, "Two Case Histories" offers three writing samples. Exhibit 7–1 illustrates the spontaneous writing of a stage 1 Alzheimer's client who benefited from the Level I writing lesson. Exhibits 7–2A and 7–2B illustrate the same client's writing in stage 2. Using the writing lesson found in Level II, this man was able to write his name and the names of several other persons who were close to him. The case history of Sara, also found in Unit 7, illustrates how other lessons that make use of the same format may be developed.

DETERMINING THE LENGTH OF THE THERAPY SESSION

Although the therapist may encounter some early-stage dementia clients who are able to tolerate 50 minutes of therapy without a break, most require shorter sessions. The lowered tolerance for sustained effort may be due as much to the pressure placed on the client by the tasks presented as to the deficits caused by the dementia. Dividing therapy into short intervals of work interspersed with a brief rest or time to chat is more effective than insisting on a full period of work.

How much work time can a given client tolerate? Since no two clients are identical, the therapist must determine the answer to this question at the initial interview. Clients at Level II may not be able to tolerate more than 20 to 30 minutes of therapy. This time should be divided into short work periods, followed by a change, followed by a repetition of the lesson.

Regardless of how much time a therapy session may consume, it is most important for the therapist to establish good rapport with both the client and the caregiver and to form a bond of trust. Many dementia clients are suspicious, placing the burden of proof of trustworthiness on the therapist. Many dementia clients are willing to try over and over again once they feel secure with the therapist; for example, one client told the therapist "I don't feel like a fool when I mess up and you're there."

Finally, less is more. A brief statement should be offered about how the lesson will help the client, such as "John, this will help you write to your son." The therapist should explain each step of the lesson at the time it is executed with a simple statement such as "We will practice using a pencil." Only information that is needed to complete a given step should be offered; for example, the therapist might say "John, pick up the pencil." The therapist should maintain eye contact, use the client's name when addressing him or her, and use as few words as possible (but repeat if repetition is needed).

SUMMARY

To use the lessons effectively

1. Inform the caregiver that he or she is expected to be present at each lesson and is expected to reinforce the lesson away from the treatment site; make certain that the caregiver understands that the lesson is incorporated into client and caregiver activities and does not require time set aside for practice.
2. Determine the client's current level of functioning according to the description under Functional Ability at the beginning of each level.
3. Choose the lesson or lessons that best suit the client's current lifestyle, activities, and needs.
4. Read the lesson to be used and the lessons in the levels that follow; reviewing lessons at all levels gives the therapist alternate strategies to use and presents a clear picture of what to do when current strategies are no longer adequate.
5. Gather all materials in advance; materials may be purchased or made by the therapist (see Appendixes B and C for a complete description of materials, how to purchase or make them, and a list of all items used).
6. Follow each step in the lesson; do not skip any steps even if the client is able to do the task without difficulty.
7. Include the caregiver in the lesson.
8. Review Part III, "Suggestions for the Health Care Professional," for additional suggestions.

Lesson Plans

LEVEL I

Functional Ability

In the early stage of Alzheimer's disease, the client's appearance and behavior are normal. The cognitive deficit may appear to be only subjective. The caregiver may notice that the individual has a tendency to forget where things are placed and to miss appointments. At the office, coworkers may have to take over some of the client's work load. At home, the individual may forget to prepare dinner or straighten the house. There may be a decrease in ability to handle finances and marketing.

When working with the client, the therapist may note some or all of the following symptoms.

Speech and language:	In conversation, language appears to be intact.
	Upon testing, there may be
	• mild naming deficit
	• poor list generation
	• some discourse incoherence
	• some perseverative responses
	• repetition difficulty only on long sentences with words that have a low probability of occurrence
	• good pragmatics (eye contact, social behavior).
Cognitive tasks:	The client still functions independently but needs to be reminded what to do. The client has noticeable difficulty learning new tasks.

Abstraction, the ability to understand and use information, is still good, but client needs a great deal of time to process information.

The client has difficulty with complex information.

The client displays concrete concept formation (is very literal) and has difficulty changing set (shifting from one task to another, e.g., spelling words to naming objects).

Orientation: The client shows intermittent or consistent confusion to place and time.

Number concepts: The client has difficulty with numbers, but can still do basic addition and subtraction.

Memory: The client shows memory loss for short-term events.

Additional observations: Although the client is physically and socially intact, there may be

- lack of initiative
- concentration deficit
- over-reaction to events
- lack of spontaneity
- feelings of "losing control"
- hostile behavior
- decline in job performance
- decreased knowledge of current events
- some deficit in memory of personal history
- flattening of affect and withdrawal from challenging situations.

LESSON ONE: WRITING A BRIEF NOTE

Description of the Lesson

Loss of the social network increases markedly as dementia progresses. Writing notes and sending cards are ways to help maintain contact with others. This lesson aims at establishing a routine to help the dementia client maintain contact with significant others while remaining oriented to current happenings.

Goal

To enable the client to write a brief letter or note to a family member, relative, or close friend.

Objectives

- To improve writing skills
- To recall recent events
- To recall names of family, friends, and others
- To improve reading skills
- To maintain social contacts

Materials

- Easy-grip or chubby dark pencil
- Paper with wide lines
- Picture of person to whom note is being written
- Picture of event (if available)
- Picture pocket
- Blank peel-off labels

Preparation

Tell the caregiver the goal of the lesson. Ask the caregiver to bring in a picture of a close relative, friend, or self to be the subject of the letter. If a special event has occurred, ask the caregiver to bring in a picture of the event (if available).

COMMENTS	INSTRUCTIONS
	9. Ask the client to put the label on the picture. Demonstrate if necessary.

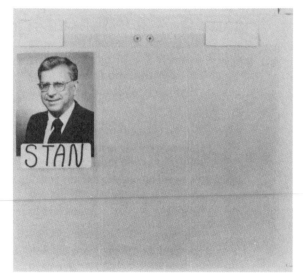

Figure 8–2 A label identifying the person in the picture has been placed on the picture.

10. If the caregiver has supplied a picture of an event or item (for example, a wedding or the purchase of a new car), show this picture to the client and say, "Tell me what you did here" (or "What is this?"). If necessary, have the caregiver assist with details.

COMMENTS	INSTRUCTIONS
The space is meant to act as a reminder that the person and event are separate. When the client was at, or part of, the event in the picture, do not space the pictures.	11. Place the picture in the picture pocket; leave a space between the two pictures.

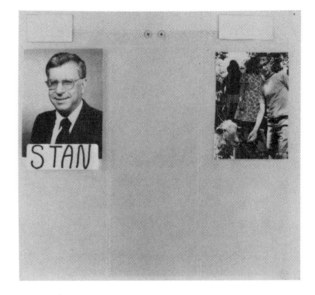

Figure 8–3 An action picture has been added to the first picture.

12. Use one or two words to identify the event picture (for example, "Fred's party" or "my dog") and ask the client to write the word(s) on a sheet of paper. If response is correct, go to Task 14. $— \rightarrow — \rightarrow — \rightarrow — \rightarrow —$

13. If incorrect, ask the caregiver to write the response.

COMMENTS	INSTRUCTIONS
	14. Give the client the pencil and ask him or her to write or copy the word(s) on a label.
	15. Ask the client to put the label on the picture. Demonstrate if necessary.

Activity Break

Compliment the client on his or her performance. Inquire about the person in the picture. Gather some information about the topic to be used in the note.

Step B

Tasks

1. Hand the client the pencil and say, "We are ready to write a short note to _____."

Direct the client's attention to the pictures and labels by pointing and looking at them.

2. Place the pictures in front of the client and say, "Try to write a note to _____ about _____."

3. If the note is correct, have the client read it aloud. End the lesson by congratulating the client and asking the client and caregiver to practice writing short notes at home.

4. If the note contains errors, print three or four short sentences for the client to copy.

5. Ask the client to read the sentences aloud.

6. Ask the client to practice writing or copying short notes at home and reading them aloud. Exhibit 8-1 is an example of a note written by an individual in stage 1.

Exhibit 8–1 Steve's Letter (Stage 1)

Steve

October – 30 1981
It is 8:30 a m – – Fridy
   I find myself smooking too much this
morning
I have to conentrate on cutting down
   on smoking

   sorry but I just cant seem to
write this morning. I will try again Tonight

I am so greatful to my wife for her
helping me thru me so much

   I am so thankfull for my wife

   I woud be lost with out her
help and he palence and love she
has shown me

Caregiver's Instructions

1. Give all materials to the caregiver.
2. Ask the caregiver to try to set aside the same time each day for the client to practice writing a note.
3. The caregiver may have the client copy the same note to the same person at each session.
4. If the client is capable of more complex work, the caregiver may have him or her write a short note on a different topic to the same person each day.
5. Remind the caregiver to use the pictures as prompts even if they are not needed. This will establish a pattern for later use.
6. When the pictures are not in use, instruct the caregiver to keep the picture pocket where it can be seen by the client and others for use as a reminder (reality orientation).

LESSON TWO: ESTABLISHING A DAILY ROUTINE

Description of the Lesson

It is important throughout the course of a dementing disease for the therapist to establish and maintain a simple, orderly routine for the client to follow. Establishing the routine early in the illness will help the client to function better in both early and late stages by reducing the need to learn new cues.

In this lesson, the therapist introduces items used by the client at home along with materials developed specifically for the lesson. The client and caregiver will use the items and materials for cueing the client's actions. The therapist will also help the client and caregiver to establish a daily routine using these cues.

Note

This is an excellent lesson for home care.

Goal

To enable the client to function independently by establishing a suitable daily routine.

Objectives

- To improve naming skills
- To improve visual recognition of objects
- To improve word recognition
- To improve picture identification

Materials

- Four to six items used for grooming that are always stored in the same location (for example, on the bathroom sink, in the medicine chest, or on a shelf). Recommended items include toothbrush, razor, comb, brush, soap, wash cloth, deodorant, morning medication (if the client is responsible for taking his or her own medication).
- Cards with peel-off pictures of items used during the lesson
- Cards with matching peel-off printed words
- Cards illustrating the use of the items
- Large blank cards
- Two sets of cards will be needed for home use

Preparation

If possible, the therapist should contact the caregiver to explain the purpose of the lesson and to arrange for him or her to bring specific personal items, such as a toothbrush or razor, from home. (It is recommended that the therapist suggest the use of an electric razor for safety purposes. The therapist may need to explain that, although at the present time the client is quite capable of using a standard razor, as the disease progresses this type of razor can be difficult and dangerous to manage.) If the caregiver does not bring items, the therapist provides items that are likely to be used at the same time (such as morning or evening) and in one specific place (such as the bathroom or kitchen).

COMMENTS	INSTRUCTIONS

Preliminary

Reality Orientation

| The client is oriented to person, place, and time. | 1. Greet the client and caregiver by name and show them into the therapy room. Example: "Good morning, Mrs. S. I'm Jane Doe, the (your title). It's nice to see you and Mr. S. Let's go into the therapy room." |
| Instructions are concrete and offer no choices. | 2. Upon entering the therapy room, instruct the caregiver and client to be seated together opposite you or to your left; therapy materials should be on a table near you but in clear view and within easy reach of everyone. Ask the caregiver for any personal items brought from home and proceed to Step A. |

Step A

Tasks

| Address the client directly and by name. | 1. Introduce the lesson. Example: "Mrs. S., I am going to help you set up a daily routine. This will help you remember what to do in the morning." |

COMMENTS	INSTRUCTIONS
	2. Give the client one of the items (for example, the toothbrush).
	3. Ask the client to identify the item.
	4. If the client names the item correctly, ask him or her to explain or demonstrate the item's function. The client may hold the item.
	5. If the client does not name the item correctly but explains or demonstrates its function correctly, cue by saying, "I brush my teeth with a _____."
	6. Once the item is identified correctly, have the client handle it and talk about its function.
	7. Take the item and put it on the table in front of the client.

Activity Break

Compliment the client on his or her efforts.

Step B

Tasks

COMMENTS	INSTRUCTIONS
The level of difficulty of these tasks depends on the number of pictures shown at one time.	1. Place four pictures (or fewer) on the table and ask the client and caregiver to look at them.
	2. Touch each picture and ask the client, "Which one is a toothbrush?"
	3. If correct, go to Task 5. If incorrect, remove two pictures. Touch each picture and ask, "Which one is a toothbrush?"

COMMENTS	INSTRUCTIONS
	4. If incorrect, ask the caregiver for the correct response and ask the client to repeat the response. For the rest of the lesson use no more than two cards at a time.
	5. Place the correct picture next to a large blank card. Ask the client to peel off the picture and place it on the blank card. Demonstrate if necessary.
	6. Place the picture beside the object.

Step C

Tasks

1. Place four word cards (or fewer) on the table and ask the client and caregiver to look at the cards.

The picture-word cards that will be used in Step D have now been created.

2. Proceed in the same manner as Step B using the word cards. In Task 5, place the word card next to the picture card and ask the client to peel the printed word off the card and place it on the picture card. Demonstrate if necessary.

Activity Break

Compliment the client on his or her efforts.

Step D

Tasks

1. Place four function cards (or fewer) on the table and ask the client and caregiver to look at them.

2. Give the client one picture-word card.

COMMENTS	INSTRUCTIONS
	3. Ask the client to match the picture-word card with the function card. If necessary, cue the client by identifying the picture-word card.
	4. Ask the client to peel off the function picture and place it on the picture-word card. Demonstrate if necessary.
	5. Hold up the picture-word function card.
	6. Point to the word and ask the client to read it.
	7. Point to the picture and say, "This is a toothbrush."
	8. Point to the function picture and say, "This is what we do with a toothbrush."
	9. Hand the client the toothbrush and say, "Show me what you do with the toothbrush."

Activity Break

Compliment the client and caregiver.

Step E

Tasks

COMMENTS	INSTRUCTIONS
All the steps are to be completed using one item before going on to the next item.	1. Tell the caregiver that he or she will give the client the next item. Reassure the caregiver that you will assist.
	2. Hand the next item to the caregiver and repeat Step A through Step D.
	3. Repeat until all items are used or the client is fatigued.

Caregiver's Instructions

1. Return the items brought in by the caregiver.
2. Give the caregiver both sets of cards with matching pictures, words, and function pictures.
3. Instruct the caregiver to post one set of picture-word function cards where the items are located and used (for example, beside the bathroom sink if soap and toothbrush are kept on the sink; beside the medicine chest or on the mirror if the razor is kept there). This set is to serve as a reminder to the client to brush his or her teeth, shave, and so forth.
4. Practice should be part of the daily routine. For example, the client is asked to identify his or her toothbrush and then is asked to point to the picture before brushing.
5. If the caregiver wishes, the second set of picture-word function cards is to be used for practicing once a day with items as instructed in the lesson.

LESSON THREE: REMEMBERING APPOINTMENTS

Description of the Lesson

In this lesson, the client and caregiver will learn to use assistive devices to aid the client in remembering appointments and special events.

Note

This is an excellent lesson for home care.

Goal

To enable the client to function independently by using a magnetic Reality Board.

Objectives

- To improve reading skills (short phrases)
- To improve time concept
- To improve visual recognition
- To maintain orientation

*Materials

- Large magnetic Reality Board*
- Magnetic labels*
- Picture of the therapist
- Small magnets to hold the picture*
- Magnetic clock*
- Stand-up clock
- Magnetic clock hands and numbers*
- Magnetic letters*

Note: * indicates materials that are part of the magnetic Message Center. For a complete description of all materials, see Appendix B.

COMMENTS	INSTRUCTIONS

Preliminary

Reality Orientation

The client is oriented to person, place, and time.	1. Greet the client and caregiver by name and show them into the therapy room. Example: "Good morning, Mrs. S. I'm Jane Doe, the (your title). It's nice to see you and Mr. S. Let's go into the therapy room."
Instructions are concrete and offer no choices.	2. Upon entering the therapy room, instruct the caregiver and client to be seated together opposite you or to your left; therapy materials should be on a table near you but in clear view and within easy reach of everyone.

Step A

Tasks

Address the client directly and by name.	1. Introduce the lesson. Example: "Mrs. S., we will practice using some things that will help you remember your appointments."
	2. Place the magnetic Reality Board within easy reach of the client. Place magnetic labels for days of the week before the client and caregiver.
	3. Point to one label at a time and ask the client to read it.
	4. Place the "Today is" label on the board and read it aloud.
	5. Touch the label and ask the client to find the label for the correct day to put next to it. If the response is correct, go to *Activity Break.* $— \rightarrow — \rightarrow — \rightarrow — \rightarrow —$ $\downarrow$

COMMENTS	INSTRUCTIONS
	6. If the response is correct but oral only, point to the labels for the days of the week and say, "Find the one that says _____." If the response is correct, go to Task 8.
	7. If the response is incorrect, point to the correct label and say, "Today is _____."
	8. Ask the client to place the label on the magnetic Reality Board. Demonstrate if necessary.

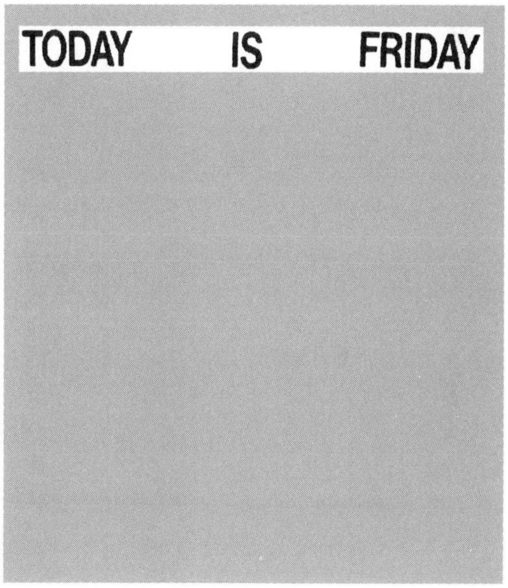

TODAY   IS   FRIDAY

Figure 8–4 The magnetic Reality Board showing the day of the week.

Activity Break

At this point, you may wish to give the caregiver additional information regarding the use of the labels to keep the client oriented.

Congratulate the client for placing the correct label on the board and say, "We will now set up the time."

COMMENTS	**INSTRUCTIONS**

Step B

1. Leave the magnetic Reality Board intact. Remove the day labels from the table.

2. Place the magnetic clock on the board without hands but with the numbers in place.

3. Set up the stand-up clock.

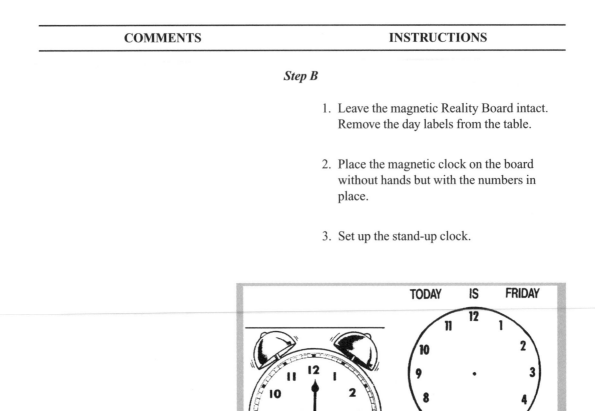

Figure 8–5 Set-up of magnetic clock without hands.

Tasks

The correct answer to Task 1 is not critical; any close approximation will do.

1. Ask whether the client or caregiver knows the correct time.

2. Set the hands of the stand-up clock to the time given and show it to the client and caregiver.

COMMENTS	INSTRUCTIONS
	3. Show the client and caregiver the hands of the magnetic clock and demonstrate setting the time.
	4. Give the magnetic clock hands first to the caregiver to try and then to the client.
	5. Remove the hands of the magnetic clock.
	6. Show the client the stand-up clock. Give the client the hands of the magnetic clock and say, "I want you to make this clock (point to the magnetic clock) have the same time as this one (point to the stand-up clock)."
	7. If the client cannot match the time, ask the caregiver to do so; then have the client try again.
	8. Say to the client, "What time is it?"
	9. Have the caregiver correct an incorrect response.
The client must be able to tell whether both clocks show the same time without help.	10. Reset the hands of both clocks and ask the client whether they are the same or different.
	11. Point out the "Today is _____" label on the magnet board, then point to the clock and say, "It is _____ o'clock."

Activity Break

Compliment the client and caregiver and tell them that there is one remaining step.

Step C

If the lesson is too long for the client, this step may be omitted but should be used at another session.	1. Remove the stand-up clock. Leave the "Today is _____" label and the clock on the board.

COMMENTS	INSTRUCTIONS
	Tasks
	1. Show the client and caregiver your picture. Ask the client who is in the picture.
	2. Using small magnets, place the picture on the magnetic Reality Board.
Do not give the client more than one or two extra letters, even if he or she is functioning at a high cognitive level.	3. Give the client magnetic letters spelling your first name.
	4. Ask the client to place the letters of your name under the picture.
	5. Have the caregiver correct if necessary.
	6. Point out the completed message: "Today is _____. It is _____ o'clock." Touch your name and add, "_____ is your therapist."

Figure 8–6 The magnetic Reality Board with the completed message.

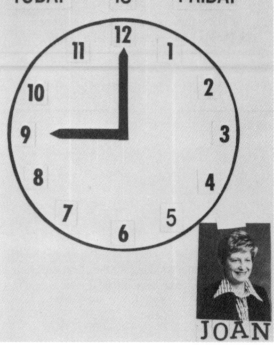

COMMENTS	INSTRUCTIONS

Activity Break

If the caregiver wishes to use magnetic messages, suggest posting them on the refrigerator.

Compliment the client and caregiver. Explain to the client and caregiver that the same technique can be used at home to remind the client of an appointment. Example: The client can use a picture of a person, plus the time, plus letters to make up a message such as "Mary, 12 o'clock, lunch, today."

Caregiver's Instructions

1. If the caregiver has acquired a magnetic Message Center, he or she is to place the clock in a permanent place where it will be readily seen. The refrigerator can be used instead of the large board. Other materials should be kept in easy reach.
2. Using as few magnetic pieces as possible to make up a clear message, the caregiver is to leave a message for the client. For a client functioning on a high cognitive level, this message may involve a direction, such as the telephone (picture of telephone and number) plus John (picture and name) plus the time (clock).
3. A client functioning at a low cognitive level may need a message saying, for example, "John is working" or "John will be home at 5 o'clock."
4. If the caregiver does not have access to magnets, he or she can leave messages by taping a large sheet of paper on any hard surface and writing with a black marking pen. Pictures can be held in place with a small piece of tape.

LESSON FOUR: PREPARING A SHOPPING LIST

Description of the Lesson

In this lesson, the client, with the assistance of the caregiver, will prepare a grocery shopping list and learn to use external aids to help focus and maintain concentration. This lesson also may be used as an initial session for discovery purposes.

Goal

To enable the client to participate actively in the daily routine of running a household by improving his or her ability to prepare a grocery list.

Objectives

- To improve list generation skills
- To improve naming skills
- To enhance memory
- To enhance writing skills
- To improve reading of single words

Materials

- Two blank shopping lists
- Individual peel-off printed words for shopping list
- Matching peel-off picture labels
- Fine-line marking pen or dark pencil
- Large and small blank cards

COMMENTS	INSTRUCTIONS

Preliminary

Reality Orientation

Client is oriented to person, place, and time.	1. Greet the client and caregiver by name and show them into the therapy room. Example: "Good morning, Mrs. S. I'm Jane Doe, the (your title). It's nice to see you and Mr. S. Let's go into the therapy room."
Instructions are concrete and offer no choices.	2. Upon entering the therapy room, instruct the caregiver and client to be seated together opposite you or to your left; therapy materials should be on a table near you but in clear view and within easy reach of everyone.

Step A

Tasks

Address the client directly and by name.	1. Introduce the lesson. Example: "Mrs. S., today I am going to teach you how to prepare a shopping list. This will help you when you go to the store to buy groceries. Mr. S. will work with us."
Use the client's list when working with him or her; your list is for reference only. Use additional sheets of lined paper or list forms as needed.	2. Place a blank shopping list between the client and the caregiver. A second blank list is for you to use as a duplicate copy and for reference during the lesson.
Task 3 is the most difficult. The caregiver may be asked to start the list as a cue. If the client cannot generate information, start the lesson at Step B.	3. Ask the client to name some items he or she might buy at the supermarket.
	4. List these items on your list.

COMMENTS	INSTRUCTIONS

5. When the client has named some items, repeat one item at a time and ask the client to write the word on his or her shopping list.

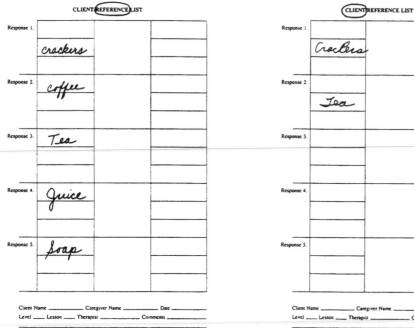

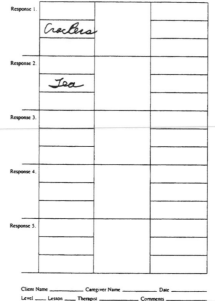

Figure 8–7 The therapist's list and the client's list shown during Task 5.

6. If the client is unable to write a word without assistance, print the word on a blank sheet of paper and instruct the client to copy the word onto his or her list. For the next incorrect word, ask the caregiver to print the word for the client and have the client copy it. Example: "Mr. S., would you print (word) for Mrs. S. and ask her to copy it?"

7. Continue until all items have been written or copied onto the client's list.

COMMENTS	INSTRUCTIONS

Activity Break

Compliment the client and caregiver. Ask if there are any questions.

Step B

Tasks

1. Offer the client a category, such as food, and ask him or her to name some items in that category.

If the client has completed Step A, list only new items.

2. List these new items on your reference list.

If the client has completed Step A, ask him or her to write new words only.

3. After the reference list has been generated, read one item at a time and ask the client to write the item on his or her list.

4. If the client is unable to write an item without assistance, print the word on a blank sheet of paper and instruct the client to copy it. For the next incorrect item, ask the caregiver to print the word and have the client copy it.

Activity Break

Compliment the client and caregiver. Show them the list they generated. Ask if there are any questions.

Step C

All notes, unless otherwise stated, should be made on the reference list.

1. Review the client's list and select available matching printed words. Place the printed words on individual cards. Note missing words.

COMMENTS	INSTRUCTIONS

Tasks

These instructions teach the caregiver how to have the client follow a complex direction. This action takes on greater significance in the later stages of the disease.

1. Give the client a word card and ask him or her to read the word.

2. Ask the client to find the matching word on his or her list. If the client does not respond correctly, go to Task 6.

3. Ask the client to peel the printed label off the card. Demonstrate if necessary.

4. Ask the client to put the printed label on top of the written word on his or her list. If necessary, point to the word or demonstrate.

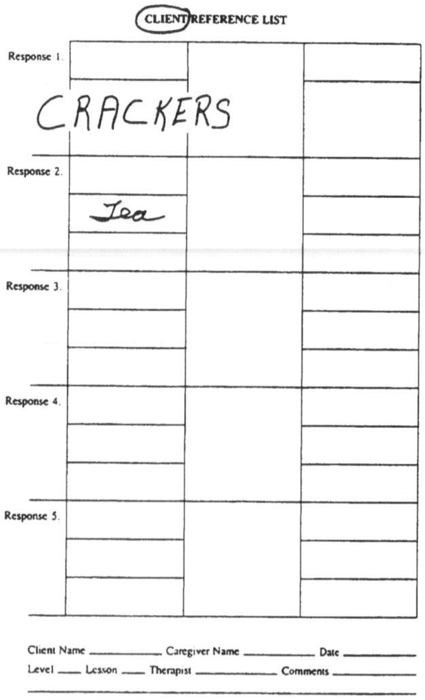

CLIENT REFERENCE LIST

Response 1.

CRACKERS

Response 2.

Tea

Response 3.

Response 4.

Response 5.

Client Name _____ Caregiver Name _____ Date _____
Level ____ Lesson ____ Therapist _____ Comments _____

Figure 8–8 The client has followed the direction in Task 4 and placed the printed label in the correct position.

COMMENTS	INSTRUCTIONS
	5. Repeat Tasks 1 through 4 until all words are used. Go to the *Activity Break* and then go to Step D.
	6. Place the word card next to the list. Point to three words on the list and ask, "Which one says _____?" If the client's response is incorrect, go to Task 8.
	7. Do Tasks 3 and 4. Repeat from Task 6 until all word cards are used. Go to *Activity Break*.
	8. If the client cannot do Task 6, point to the correct word and ask, "Does this say _____?" Have the caregiver correct the response or validate the client's response.
	9. Do Tasks 3 and 4. Repeat from Task 8 until all word cards are used. Go to *Activity Break*.

Activity Break

Compliment the client and caregiver and explain that one more step remains. Stress the importance of going through all the steps.

Step D

COMMENTS	INSTRUCTIONS
All notes, unless otherwise stated, should be made on the reference list.	1. Check the pictures to ensure that all items on the client's list are present. Note pictures that are missing. Select pictures that are on the client's list and place them on large blank cards, with no more than four to a card.

Tasks

1. Show the client a set of pictures and ask him or her to identify the items. If the client cannot name an item or circumlocutes,

COMMENTS	INSTRUCTIONS

provide a cue. If necessary, name the item and ask the client to repeat.

2. Remove one picture from the set and place it on a small card.

This task becomes increasingly difficult to follow as the disease progresses.

3. Give the client the small card and ask him or her to match the picture to the printed label on the list. If the response is incorrect, go to Task 6. — → — → — → — → — → —

→ 4. Ask the client to peel the picture off the card.

5. Ask the client to put the picture next to the printed label on his or her list. If necessary, point to the label or demonstrate. If response is correct, repeat until all the pictures and labels are matched. Go to *Activity Break.*

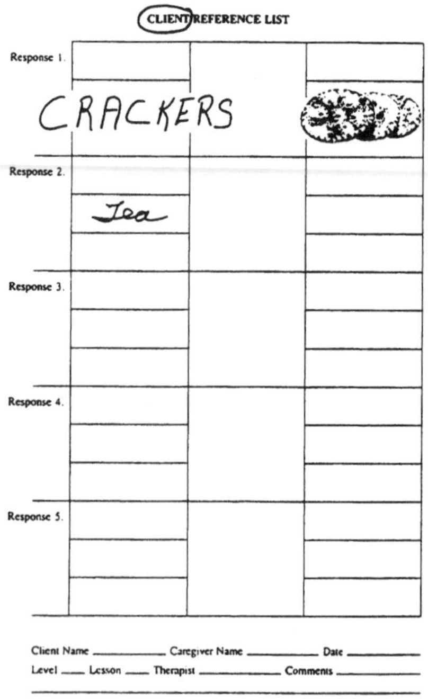

CLIENT REFERENCE LIST

Response 1.

CRACKERS

Response 2.

Tea

Response 3.

Response 4.

Response 5.

Client Name _____ Caregiver Name _____ Date _____
Level ____ Lesson ____ Therapist _____ Comments _____

Figure 8–9 The client's list illustrating the correct placement of the labels and pictures.

COMMENTS	INSTRUCTIONS

6. Place the picture next to the client's list, ← — ↓ point to three words on the list and ask, "Which one says _____?"

7. Do Tasks 4 and 5. Repeat from Task 6 until all the pictures and words are matched. Go to *Activity Break*.

Activity Break

Congratulate the client and caregiver and say, "Now I will give you some cards to use at home. Bring them with you next time you come." Remove the words and pictures and place them on individual cards. Date the client's list and your reference list and place them in the client's file. Give the caregiver the cards, a blank shopping list, and instructions for home sessions. Stress the importance of reinforcement at home.

Caregiver's Instructions

1. Instruct the caregiver to work with the client at home to generate an actual shopping list. Stress that the list can be short—three to five items are sufficient.
2. Suggest that both the client and the caregiver look in the refrigerator or cupboard for items to put on the list.
3. The caregiver should ask the client to name the items and to write or copy the words onto the shopping list.
4. The caregiver and client should then match the words and pictures from the previous session to the items on their new shopping list.
5. If they do not have a picture, they should try to find one in a magazine and cut it out.
6. Instruct the caregiver to bring a completed shopping list to the next session.
7. The caregiver is responsible for caring for all materials and for bringing them to the next session.

LESSON FIVE: USING THE SHOPPING LIST

Description of the Lesson

The client, with the aid of the caregiver, matches items on a prepared shopping list with simulated grocery items, printed labels, and pictures.

Goal

To enable the client to participate actively in the daily routine of running a household by assisting in shopping for groceries.

Objectives

- To improve list generation skills
- To improve naming skills
- To enhance memory
- To enhance writing skills
- To improve reading of single words

Materials

- Shopping lists
- Basket or box for simulated grocery items
- Four or more simulated grocery items
- Printed peel-off grocery labels
- Matching peel-off pictures
- Fine-line marking pen or dark pencil
- Blank lined paper

Preparation

If the client and caregiver have completed Lesson 4, choose simulated grocery items from the list generated at that lesson. If they have not completed Lesson 4, prepare a short list for use during this lesson. Complete the *Preliminary* section and start at Step B.

COMMENTS	INSTRUCTIONS

Preliminary

Reality Orientation

Tasks

Client is oriented to person, place, and time.	1. Greet the client and caregiver by name and show them into the therapy room. Example: "Good morning, Mrs. S. I'm Jane Doe, the (your title). It's nice to see you and Mr. S. Let's go into the therapy room."
Instructions are concrete and offer no choices.	2. Upon entering the therapy room, instruct the caregiver and client to be seated together opposite you or to your left; therapy materials should be on a table near you but in clear view and within easy reach of everyone.
Address the client directly and by name.	3. Introduce the lesson. Example: "Mrs. S., we are going to practice using a shopping list."

Step A

Tasks

These tasks are designed to include the caregiver early in the lesson.	1. Ask the caregiver for the shopping list. Example: "Mr. S., may I have the shopping list you and Mrs. S. made?"
Use the client's list when working with him or her; your list is for reference only.	2. Check the items on the client's list against those on your reference list; add new items to your list and note them.
Task 3 is the most difficult.	3. Ask the client to name items to be purchased. Example: "Mrs. S., tell me some of the things you plan to buy at the store."

COMMENTS	INSTRUCTIONS
If cues are needed, the caregiver should be encouraged to give them.	4. If the client is unable to respond correctly, cue. Example: "Let's start with something you drink at breakfast."
Note which method of cueing works best.	5. If verbal cueing is not sufficient, show the client four pictures at a time and ask which ones might be on the list.
	6. If cueing does not work, let the client see the list. Ask the caregiver to read items on list.

Activity Break

Admit to the difficulty of the task and praise the client's efforts as you make your notes. Go to Step C.

Step B

Tasks

Include the caregiver as an active participant.	1. Inform the caregiver and client that they need a short shopping list with which to practice.
	2. Ask the client to name some items that he or she might buy at the supermarket. If necessary, allow the caregiver to assist.
Make all notations on your reference list.	3. Write these items on a sheet of lined paper; this will be your reference list. Make a copy of this list for the client to use.

Step C

Tasks

Step C reinforces Step A (or Step B) and helps the client with writing skills.	1. Give the list to the client and ask him or her to read the items.

COMMENTS	INSTRUCTIONS
	2. Turn the list over so that the client cannot see the items.
	3. Place a sheet of lined paper before the client. Tell the client that you will say each item on the list and that he or she is to write the word on the paper.
	4. If the client is unable to write a word, print the word and instruct the client to copy it. At the next error, instruct the caregiver to print the word for the client and have the client copy it. Example: "Mr. S., would you print (word) for Mrs. S. and ask her to copy it?"
	5. Write the client's name and date on the paper and place it in the client's file.

Activity Break

Compliment the client and caregiver.

Step D

Tasks

COMMENTS	INSTRUCTIONS
Without additional cueing this task is difficult. The more pictures presented at one time, the more difficult the task. Start by presenting no more than two pictures at a time. Increase or decrease the number of pictures according to the client's ability. It may be necessary to present one picture at a time.	1. Place the client's list before the client and caregiver. Show them a group of pictures and ask the client to match the pictures to the items on his or her list. Example: "Look at these pictures and tell me which ones are on your shopping list."
	2. If necessary, cue the client. Example: Point to a picture and ask, "Do you have _____ on your list?" Point to a picture and say, "Find _____ on this list." Point to the list.

COMMENTS	INSTRUCTIONS
	3. Ask the client to peel the picture off the sheet and place it on a blank card. Demonstrate if necessary.
	4. Place the matching printed label under the picture on the card and ask the client to read it.
	5. Repeat until each item on the shopping list has a corresponding card.

Activity Break

Compliment the client and caregiver. Tell them there is one more step to complete.

Step E

Tasks

COMMENTS	INSTRUCTIONS
	1. Place the previously prepared grocery items where they can be seen and reached with ease.
	2. Give the caregiver the cards.
	3. Give the client a basket or box.
Presenting the direction to the caregiver in this task will give you a chance to observe the spontaneous interaction between the pair.	4. Tell the caregiver, "We are going to pretend that you are at the store. I want you to give Mrs. S. one card and ask her to find the item."
	5. If the client's response is correct, have the client place the item in the basket and repeat Task 4 until all items are in the basket.
	6. If the client's response is incorrect, have the caregiver hand the client the item and name the item.

COMMENTS	INSTRUCTIONS
	7. Have the client put the item in the basket. Demonstrate if necessary.

Activity Break

When all items are in the basket, congratulate the client and caregiver on their teamwork and tell them that they are to try matching items at the supermarket with the items on the cards.

Caregiver's Instructions

1. Return the shopping list and the matching picture-word cards to the caregiver.
2. Instruct the caregiver to have the client match the items at the supermarket with the ones on the shopping list.
3. Upon returning from the supermarket, the client is to match the items on the list with the ones purchased.
4. The caregiver and client prepare a new list for the next session.

Note: For suggestions on how to have a successful shopping trip, see the section on *Helpful Hints* in Unit 12.

LESSON SIX: UNPACKING THE GROCERIES

Description of the Lesson

The client and caregiver learn how to use external devices (labels and pictures) as assistive devices in remembering household items and their location. This lesson may be carried out either in an ADL room or in the client's home.

Goal

To enable the client to participate actively in the daily routine of running a household by unpacking and storing purchased items.

Objectives

- To improve naming skills
- To improve reading skills
- To improve recognition skills

Materials

- Bag or box of groceries
- List of grocery items (shopping list)
- Matching peel-off labels
- Matching peel-off pictures
- Marking pencil
- Blank lined paper
- Clip board

Site Adaptations

If the lesson is to take place in the ADL room, before the arrival of the client and caregiver set the bag or box of groceries on the kitchen table. Place a written list of the items and matching labels and pictures at your place.

If the lesson is to take place in the client's home, instruct the caregiver about how to adapt the kitchen in advance. The caregiver is to have one bag of groceries on the kitchen table ready for your arrival. The bag should contain only items agreed upon in advance. The caregiver should make a list of these items for your use. Ask the caregiver to leave space on the table for the list, matching labels, and pictures. If the caregiver does not have labels and pictures, bring these materials.

COMMENTS	INSTRUCTIONS

Preliminary

Reality Orientation

The client is oriented to person, place, and time.	1. Greet the client and caregiver by name. Example: "Good morning, Mrs. S. I'm Jane Doe, the (your title). It's nice to see you and Mr. S. Welcome to our activities room" (or, "I'm happy to be at your house").
The information presented is simple and concrete. Time is allowed between your comments for the client to respond.	2. Identify the exact location of the action and the action itself. Example: "We will work in the kitchen. We will unpack groceries."
Include the caregiver in the remarks.	3. Specify the purpose of the action. Example: "This will help you and Mr. S. remember what is in your cupboards."
	4. Instruct the client and caregiver to be seated at the table.
	5. If you are at the client's home, ask the caregiver for the shopping list and other materials.

Step A

Tasks

	1. Describe the action as you begin. Example: Place the shopping list between the client and the caregiver and say, "We are going to match the groceries in the bag to the ones on this list."
Allow the client to hold the item if he or she wishes.	2. Take one item out of the bag. Show it to the client and say, "Tell me what this is." If the client is unable to name item, allow him or her to read the label.

COMMENTS	INSTRUCTIONS
	3. Have the client match the item with items on the shopping list. Ask the caregiver to check the item on the list when it is located.

Step B

Tasks

COMMENTS	INSTRUCTIONS
The degree of difficulty of this task depends on the number of labels shown at one time.	1. Using the same item, show the client the matching printed label. Ask the client to match the item with the label.
	2. Ask the client to peel off the label and place it on a card. Demonstrate if necessary.

Step C

Tasks

COMMENTS	INSTRUCTIONS
The difficulty of the tasks increases with the number of pictures shown at one time.	1. Using the same item, show the client two to four pictures. Ask the client to match the item with one of the pictures.
	2. Ask the client to peel off the picture and place it on the same card with the printed label. Demonstrate if necessary.

Step D

Tasks

COMMENTS	INSTRUCTIONS
	1. Ask the caregiver to put the item on a shelf where it can be easily seen.
	2. Repeat all tasks from Step A to Step D until all items are in the cupboard.

COMMENTS	INSTRUCTIONS

Activity Break

Compliment the client and caregiver. Stress that the quantity of groceries is not important; it is going through all the steps of identification that counts. Stress teamwork.

Step E

Tasks

1. When all the items are in the cupboard, instruct the client and caregiver to join you at the cupboard.

2. Hand the client one card and ask him or her to locate the item on the shelf. If the client is unable to locate the item, ask the caregiver to help.

To be effective, the labels must be visible.

3. When the item is located, demonstrate peeling off the label and picture from the card and placing them on the shelf where the item is located. Explain the action during the demonstration. Example: "Now we put the label and picture here." After the demonstration, explain the purpose of the action to the client and caregiver. Example: "This will help you remember what belongs on this shelf."

4. Hand the client the next card and repeat Task 2.

5. Ask the client to peel off the word and picture from the card and to place them on the shelf where they can be seen. If the client is not successful, ask the caregiver to demonstrate. On the following card, ask the caregiver to help the client peel off the word and picture and put them in place.

COMMENTS	INSTRUCTIONS
	6. Repeat Step E until all the words and pictures are on the shelf.
	Activity Break
	Compliment the client and caregiver and tell them that there is one more step.

Step F

	Tasks
If the lesson is too long, do not proceed to Step F. This may be used as a separate lesson.	1. Tell the client and caregiver that you will now show them how to use the labels to prepare a new shopping list.
	2. Remove four items from the shelf
	3. Ask the client to point to an empty space on the shelf.
	4. Ask the client to name the missing item. The client may read the label.
	5. Give the client the clip board with blank paper and a pencil. Ask the client to write or copy the name of the missing item. If the client cannot write or copy the word, have him or her remove the label from the shelf and place it on the blank paper. Assist if necessary.
	6. Replace the items on the shelf. Repeat Tasks 3 through 5 until all items are identified.
	Activity Break
	Compliment the caregiver and client.

Caregiver's Instructions

If the lesson was done outside the client's home

1. Help the caregiver generate a short shopping list.
2. Using the caregiver's list, give the caregiver the matching labels and pictures.
3. Instruct the caregiver to place the list items in a bag and then to have the client place the items on the shelf in the same manner at home as in the training room.
4. The caregiver then helps the client to place the pictures and labels on the shelf where the items are located.
5. Continue with instructions listed below.

If the lesson was done in the client's home

1. Instruct the caregiver to leave the labels and pictures in place on the shelf.
2. The same item should be kept in the same place to help avoid confusion.
3. When the space is empty, the client should write or copy the item onto a sheet of paper. This paper will become the new shopping list.
4. If the client is unable to write or copy the word, the caregiver should remove the label or the picture from the shelf and place it on the sheet of paper. The caregiver should leave either the label or the picture on the shelf to remind him or her where to place the item after it is purchased.
5. The list should be placed where it can be seen, and new items should be added as needed.
6. The client should read the list aloud each day.

LEVEL II

Functional Ability

The second stage of Alzheimer's disease is characterized by a definite impairment of cognitive functioning that is most obvious for memory of recent events. No assistance is required with toileting or eating, but the client may have some difficulty dressing or choosing the proper clothing. Bathing may become a problem; the client may exhibit a fear of bathing and refuse to bathe or may do an inadequate job of cleaning or grooming.

The therapist should observe the client for the following symptoms.

Speech and language:	Although social communication remains good, the content of speech may be confused or irrelevant. Circumlocution is evident. The client "avoids the issue" and appears to have difficulty coming to the point.

Upon testing, there may be
- increased difficulty in choosing words
- intact syntax
- mild perseveration (the client may add irrelevant words at the end of a sentence)
- repetition for short, high-frequency items is spared.

Cognitive tasks:	Abstraction is obviously affected. The client functions with the aid of the caregiver. Cognitive skills are noticeably reduced.
Orientation:	Increased confusion to person, place, and time. The client's concept of time is most seriously impaired.
Number concepts:	Very poor or nonexistent.
Memory:	Increased memory deficit: the client may be unable to recall his or her address, familiar telephone numbers, or names of close members of the family.
	Memory is poor to very poor for recent events.
Additional observations:	There may be

- loss of social ability
- sleeping disorders
- difficulties with ADLs
- hallucinations
- paranoia
- lability
- wandering
- excessive passivity
- frequent repetitive behaviors.

LESSON ONE: WRITING

Description of the Lesson

Recognizing one's own name as well as the names of significant others is an important step in maintaining orientation. Many clients, even in the later stages of Alzheimer's disease, must retain the ability to sign their names. In this lesson, the client will practice writing his or her name as well as the names of two or three significant others. The client will also practice associating the written name with pictures of these persons.

Goal

To enable the client to remain oriented to person.

Objectives

- To improve copying skills
- To improve naming skills
- To improve visual recognition

Materials

- Easy-grip or chubby dark pencil
- Paper with wide lines
- Appropriate pictures
- Blank peel-off labels
- Picture pocket

Preparation

Inform the caregiver of the lesson goal. Ask the caregiver to bring pictures of people familiar to the client. Be certain to specify that group pictures are not appropriate.

COMMENTS	INSTRUCTIONS

Preliminary

Reality Orientation

Orientation to person, place, and time becomes more important as the disease progresses. These preliminary steps should never be omitted.	1. Greet the client and caregiver by name and show them into the therapy room. Example: "Good morning, Mrs. S. I'm Jane Doe, the (your title). It's nice to see you and Mr. S. Let's go into the therapy room."
Instructions are concrete and offer no choices.	2. Upon entering the therapy room, instruct the caregiver and client to be seated together opposite you or to your left; therapy materials should be on a table near you but in clear view and within easy reach of everyone. Ask the caregiver for the pictures and proceed to Step A.

Step A

Tasks

Address the client directly and by name.	1. Introduce the lesson. Example: "Mrs. S., I am going to help you with your writing. This will help you with your memory."
	2. Give the client the picture of himself or herself.
	3. Ask the client who is in the picture.
Do not use a mirror to help the client. This may cause confusion.	4. If correct, continue. If incorrect, ask the caregiver to identify the person in the picture.
	5. Place the picture in the picture pocket.
	6. Ask the client to try to write his or her name on a sheet of paper.

COMMENTS	INSTRUCTIONS
	7. If incorrect, ask the caregiver to print the correct name.
	8. Have the client write or copy his or her name on a label.
	9. Ask the client to read the name aloud.
	10. Ask the client to put the label on the picture. Demonstrate or assist if necessary.
	11. Repeat Tasks 2 through 10 using the remaining pictures.

Activity Break

Compliment the client on his or her efforts. If the client is not fatigued, the lesson may be repeated.

Caregiver's Instructions

1. Give the caregiver the picture pocket, pictures, and blank labels.
2. Instruct the caregiver to practice the lesson with the client each day.
3. The caregiver should not change pictures. If it becomes necessary to use fewer pictures at home, instruct the caregiver to use the client's picture and the caregiver's picture and to eliminate the others.
4. When not in use, the picture pocket should be placed with the pictures and labels where they can be seen by the client and used for reality orientation.

LESSON TWO: ESTABLISHING A DAILY ROUTINE

Description of the Lesson

At Level II, a simple, ordered, daily routine is vital for both client and caregiver. In this lesson the client and caregiver, using items brought from home and materials supplied by the therapist, learn how to use visual cues to help the morning routine. Before the lesson, the therapist should explain to the caregiver the purpose of the lesson and arrange to have the caregiver bring specific personal items, such as a toothbrush or razor, from home. (If the caregiver plans to bring the client's razor, the therapist should suggest the use of an electric razor for safety purposes.)

Note

This is an excellent lesson for home care.

Goal

To enable the client to participate actively in ADLs by establishing a suitable daily routine.

Objectives

- To improve naming skills
- To improve object recognition
- To improve word recognition
- To improve picture identification
- To improve task orientation

Materials

- Four to six items used for grooming that are always stored in the same location (for example, on the sink in the bathroom, in the medicine chest, or on a shelf). Recommended items include toothbrush, razor, comb, brush, soap, washcloth, deodorant, towel.
- Cards with peel-off pictures of items used during the lesson
- Cards with matching peel-off words
- Cards illustrating the use of the items
- Large blank cards
- Two sets of cards will be needed for home use.

COMMENTS	INSTRUCTIONS

Preliminary

Reality Orientation

The client is oriented to person, place, and time.

1. Greet the client and caregiver by name and show them into the therapy room. Example: "Good morning Mrs. S. I'm Jane Doe, the (your title). It's nice to see you and Mr. S. Let's go into the therapy room."

Instructions are concrete and offer no choices.

2. Upon entering the therapy room, instruct the caregiver and client to be seated together opposite you or to your left; therapy materials should be on a table near you but in clear view and within easy reach of everyone. Ask the caregiver for any personal items brought from home and proceed to Step A.

Step A

Tasks

1. Introduce the lesson. Example: "Mrs. S., I am going to help you remember what to do in the morning."

2. Give the client one of the items (for example, the toothbrush).

The client may deny not knowing what to do in the morning. If this is the case, respond by saying, for example, "Good, then this will make it even easier."

3. Ask the client to identify the item.

4. Acknowledge a correct response. If the response is incorrect, ask the caregiver to name the item and the client to repeat the name.

COMMENTS	INSTRUCTIONS
Confusion may be accepted but never ignored. Each item should be identified and the correct response given. This directive should be followed whenever confusion on the part of the client is encountered.	5. If the client appears to be confused, acknowledge the confusion and correct the response. Have the client repeat the response.
	6. Show the client two picture cards. Ask the client to point to the picture of the toothbrush. Demonstrate if necessary.
	7. Acknowledge the correct response. Correct an incorrect response.
	8. Place the picture on the large blank card.

Activity Break

Compliment the client on his or her efforts. If the client cannot read single words skip Step B and go to Step C.

Step B

Tasks

1. Leave the item and the matching picture card on the table before the client.

2. Show the client two word cards. Ask the client to point to the one that reads toothbrush. Demonstrate if necessary.

3. Acknowledge a correct response. Correct an incorrect response.

4. Peel the word off the card and place it next to the picture.

→ 5. Touch the word, the picture, and the item. Repeat the name each time.

COMMENTS	INSTRUCTIONS
	6. Repeat Task 5 with the caregiver saying the item's name.
	7. Repeat Task 5 with the client saying the item's name.

Activity Break

Compliment the client on his or her efforts. Ask the caregiver if there are any questions.

Step C

Tasks

1. Leave the picture-word card and the item on the table where they can be easily seen.

2. Place two function cards on the table before the client.

3. Ask the client to match the picture-word card with the function card. Cue the client by identifying the picture-word card. Demonstrate if necessary.

4. Peel off the function picture and place it on the picture-word card.

5. Hold up the card with the picture-word function.

6. Point to the word and ask the client to read it.

7. Point to the picture and say, "This is a toothbrush."

8. Point to the function picture and say, "This is what we do with a toothbrush."

COMMENTS	INSTRUCTIONS
	9. Hand the client the toothbrush and say, "Show me what you do with the toothbrush."

Activity Break

Compliment the client on his or her efforts. Tell the caregiver that he or she will give the client the next item. Reassure the caregiver that you will assist.

Step D

Tasks

COMMENTS	INSTRUCTIONS
Step D may require a good bit of time and patience, but it is important that the caregiver and the client be given the opportunity to work together successfully.	1. Hand the next item to the caregiver. Ask the caregiver to have the client identify the item.
	2. Present the two picture cards to the caregiver. Ask the caregiver to show the client the cards.
	3. Ask the caregiver to have the client point to the picture. Assist if necessary.
Do not become discouraged if the client is able to use only one item the first time this lesson is presented. Remember, you are training two persons. Repetition and consistency are key.	4. Continue working in this manner with the caregiver and client, repeating from Step A through Step C for each item until all items are used or the client is fatigued.

Caregiver's Instructions

1. Return all personal items, two sets of cards with matching pictures, and function pictures to the caregiver. Do not include the word cards unless the client is reading single words.

2. The caregiver is to post one set of pictures illustrating the items and pictures of the items' functions where the actual items are located and used (for example, beside the bathroom sink if soap and toothbrush are kept on the sink; beside the medicine chest or on the mirror if the razor is located there). This set of cards serves as a reminder to the client to brush his or her teeth, shave, and so forth.

3. The second set of picture-function cards is to be used for practicing once a day with items as instructed in the lesson.

LESSON THREE: REMEMBERING APPOINTMENTS

Description of the Lesson

In this lesson, the client and caregiver will learn to use assistive devices to aid the client in remembering appointments and special events.

Note

This is an excellent lesson for home care.

Goal

To enable the client to function more successfully by using an assistive magnetic board.

Objectives

- To improve visual recognition of single words
- To improve visual recognition of objects
- To improve time concept
- To improve orientation

Materials

- Large magnetic Reality Board
- Magnetic labels*
- Picture of the therapist
- Small magnets to hold the picture*
- Stand-up clock
- Magnetic clock*
- Clock hands and numbers*
- Magnetic letters*

Note: * indicates materials that are part of the magnetic Message Center. For a complete description of all materials, see Appendix B.

COMMENTS	**INSTRUCTIONS**

Preliminary

Reality Orientation

The client is oriented to person, place, and time.	1. Greet the client and caregiver by name and show them into the therapy room. Example: "Good morning, Mrs. S. I'm Jane Doe, the (your title). It's nice to see you and Mr. S. Let's go into the therapy room."
Instructions are concrete and offer no choices.	2. Upon entering the therapy room, instruct the caregiver and client to be seated together opposite you or to your left; therapy materials should be on a table near you but in clear view and within easy reach of everyone.

Step A

Tasks

1. Address the client directly and by name. Introduce the lesson. Example: "Mrs. S., we will practice using some devices that will help you remember appointments."

2. Place the magnetic board within the client's reach. Place magnetic labels for days of the week before the client and caregiver.

3. Point to one label at a time and ask the client to read it.

4. If the client cannot do so, read the label and ask the client to repeat.

COMMENTS	INSTRUCTIONS
	5. Place the "Today is" label on the board and tell the client what it says.
	6. Touch the label and ask the client, "What day is today?"
	7. If response is correct, say, "Find the label that says _____" and go to Task 8. For an incorrect response, point to the correct label and say, "Today is _____."
	8. Give the client the label.
	9. Point to the magnetic board and say, "Put the day here." Assist if necessary.

Activity Break

At this point, you may wish to give the caregiver additional information regarding the use of the labels to keep the client oriented.	Congratulate the client for placing the correct label on the board and say, "We will now work on the time."

Step B

	1. Leave the message on the magnetic board. Remove the day labels from the table.
	2. Place the magnetic clock on the board with numbers in place without hands.
	3. Set up the stand-up clock.

Tasks

The correct answer to Task 1 is not critical; any close approximation will do. The client needs only to say whether it is morning, afternoon, or night. Do not ignore an incorrect response of this type.	1. Ask whether the client or caregiver knows the correct time.
	2. Set the hands of the stand-up clock to the time given and show it to the client and caregiver.

COMMENTS	INSTRUCTIONS
	3. Set the hands of the magnetic clock to the same time as shown on the stand-up clock and ask the client whether both clocks show the same time.
The client does not have to know the time, but he or she must be able to recognize whether the clocks show the same time.	4. Repeat the task with a different time on each clock. If incorrect, go to *Activity Break*.
	5. If both responses are correct, remove the hands of the magnetic clock.
	6. Show the client the stand-up clock. Give the client the hands of the magnetic clock and say, "I want you to make this clock (point to the magnetic clock) show the same time as this one" (point to the stand-up clock). Assist if necessary. If correct, ask the client, "What time is it on the clocks?"
	7. If the client cannot match the times, go to *Activity Break*.
	8. Have the caregiver correct an incorrect response.

Activity Break

If the client was unable to match times on the clocks and was also unable to tell the time, remove the clock from the magnetic board. Point out the message on the board: "Today is
_____." If the client was able either to match the time or to tell the correct time, leave the clock on the board and say, "It is _____ o'clock." To the caregiver, say, "We will put one more piece of information on the board."

COMMENTS	INSTRUCTIONS
	Step C
	1. Remove the stand-up clock.
	2. If the client could not tell the time and was also unable to read the time, remove the magnetic clock from the board.
	Tasks
	1. Show the client and caregiver your picture. Ask the client who is in the picture.
	2. Using small magnets, place the picture on the magnetic board.
	3. Give the client magnetic letters spelling your first name.
	4. Place the letters in the correct order in front of the client.
	5. Ask the client to place the letters of your name under your picture.
	6. Have the caregiver correct if necessary.
	7. Point out the completed message: "Today is _____. We are seeing _____ at _____ o'clock."
	Activity Break
If the caregiver wishes to use magnetic messages, suggest posting them on the refrigerator.	Compliment the client and caregiver. Explain to them that the same technique can be used at home to remind the client of an appointment. Example: Using a picture of a person, plus the time, plus an action label or letters, the caregiver can formulate a message such as "Mary, 12 o'clock, lunch, today."

Caregiver's Instructions

1. If the caregiver has acquired a magnetic Message Center, he or she is to place the clock in a permanent place where it will be readily seen. The refrigerator can be used instead of the large board. Other materials should be kept in easy reach.
2. Using as few magnetic pieces as possible to make up a clear message, the caregiver is to leave a message for the client, such as "John is working" or "John will be home at 5 o'clock."
3. If the caregiver does not have access to a magnetic Message Center, he or she can leave messages by taping a large sheet of paper on any hard surface and writing with a black marking pen. Pictures can be held in place with a small piece of masking tape.

LESSON FOUR: PREPARING A SHOPPING LIST

Description of the Lesson

In this lesson the client, with the assistance of the caregiver, will participate in preparing a grocery shopping list using external aids (pictures and labels).

Goal

To enable the client to participate actively in the daily routine of running a household by participating in the preparation of a shopping list.

Objectives

- To maintain task orientation
- To reduce word-finding problems when preparing a grocery list
- To enhance memory
- To improve reading skills (nouns)
- To improve copying skills (single words)

Materials

- Two blank shopping lists
- Individual peel-off printed grocery labels (for food and cleaning items)
- Matching peel-off picture labels
- Easy-grip marker or pencil

COMMENTS	INSTRUCTIONS

Preliminary

Reality Orientation

The client is oriented to person, place, and time.	1. Greet the client and caregiver by name and show them into the therapy room. Example: "Good morning, Mrs. S. I'm Jane Doe, the (your title). It's nice to see you and Mr. S. Let's go into the therapy room."
Instructions are concrete and offer no choices.	2. Upon entering the therapy room, instruct the caregiver and client to be seated together opposite you or to your left; therapy materials should be on a table near you but in clear view and within easy reach of everyone.
Use of the client's name helps to maintain orientation and to gain and direct his or her attention to the task.	3. Introduce the lesson. Example: "Mrs. S., today we are going to prepare a shopping list. This will help when you go to the store with Mr. S."
Do not comment on this action. Use the client's list when working with him or her; your list is for reference only.	4. Place a blank shopping list between the client and caregiver. A second blank list is for you to use as a duplicate copy and for note-taking during the lesson.
When the client is in the early part of stage 2 Alzheimer's disease, it may be possible to present pictures from more than one category at the same time, ask the client to point to the one that he or she eats, and then name the object. As the disease progresses, however, it will be necessary to reduce the number of pictures and categories.	5. Select pictures from one category (for example, food).
	6. Show the pictures to the caregiver. Have the caregiver select four pictures of items that are used in the home (for example, cheese, milk, bread, and juice).
	7. Write these items on the reference list.

COMMENTS	INSTRUCTIONS

Step A

Tasks

If the client is successful using four cards, a fifth card may be added. Do not add a second category of cards until the first group is mastered.

1. Place the four pictures selected by the caregiver before the client.

2. Tell the client the category and ask him or her to repeat it. Example: "Mrs. S., these are things we eat. (Pause) Mrs. S., what are these?"

3. Touch one picture and name the item. Example: Touch the picture, pause, direct the client's gaze to the picture, and say, "Butter."

Task 4 is used for reinforcement.

4. Tell the caregiver and client to take turns repeating this task.

5. After the client has named the item, assist him or her in peeling off the picture and placing it on the client's shopping list.

6. Point to the picture on the client's list and ask the client to complete the statement "This is a(n) _____." Correct an incorrect response and have the client repeat the correct response.

7. After obtaining the correct response, state the item's function and name. Example: "We eat _____."

8. Repeat Tasks 2 through 7 until all pictures are on the client's list.

Activity Break

The client is given time to adapt to the completion of the task before a new task is attempted.

Compliment the client on the effort put forth. Ask the caregiver if there are any questions. Tell the client and the caregiver that they have completed the first part of the lesson.

COMMENTS	INSTRUCTIONS

Step B

1. Select the printed labels that match the pictures on the client's shopping list.

2. Place the labels on individual cards.

Tasks

1. To introduce the new task, show the client one card and say "Mrs. S., we are going to match the word on this card with a picture on our shopping list."

2. Ask the client to read the word on the card. If correct, congratulate the client and repeat the word. Example: "Very good, Mrs. S., the word is _____." If incorrect, ask the caregiver to read the word and the client to repeat it. Example: "Mr. S., will you read this word for Mrs. S.? Good. That's _____. Mrs. S., say _____."

The first direction is abstract; the second is concrete.

3. Ask the client to match the word on the card with a picture on the shopping list. Example: Hold the card next to the pictures on the shopping list and ask, "Mrs. S., which picture is the same as the word on this card?" If incorrect, repeat the direction using the word on the card. Example: Hold the card next to the pictures on the shopping list, point to the card, and say, "Mrs. S., this card says _____." Point to the pictures and ask, "Which one is _____?" If incorrect, supply the correct response. Example: "Mrs. S. (point to the card), the card says _____ (point to the picture), and this picture is a _____."

4. After the word and picture are matched, peel the printed label off the card and place it to the right of the picture.

COMMENTS	INSTRUCTIONS
	5. Repeat Tasks 1 through 4 until all the pictures have matching labels.

Activity Break

Compliment the client on the effort put forth. Ask the caregiver if there are any questions. Tell the client and the caregiver that they have completed the second part of the lesson.

Step C

Tasks

COMMENTS	INSTRUCTIONS
Step C may be used for discovery purposes.	1. Introduce the new task. Example: "Mrs. S., I want you to copy some words. I will help."
	2. Point to the first picture on the shopping list and say, "Mrs. S., this is _____." Pause.
	3. Point to the word to the right of the picture and say, "This says _____." Pause.
	4. Hand the pen to the client. Pointing to the space to the right of the printed word, say, "Mrs. S., copy _____."
	5. If the client does not respond, demonstrate and then hand the pen back to the client.
	6. If the client does not respond, help initiate the action by guiding the client's hand. Upon completion of the word, place the client's hand in position and say, "Try again." If there is no response, end at this point by saying, "You did well. This is quite difficult. I know you are tired. We can try again when you are ready."

COMMENTS	INSTRUCTIONS
	7. If the client is successful, repeat Tasks 2 through 6 for each picture.
All notes are to be made on the reference list unless they are needed to clarify the client's writing.	8. Collect the shopping list and write the client's name and the date at the top. Remove the pictures and labels and place them back on the cards. Write the words in the blank spaces of the shopping list.

Activity Break

Compliment the client and caregiver. Ask them if they have any questions.

Caregiver's Instructions

1. Give the caregiver a blank shopping list, four picture cards, and four matching labels. The caregiver is to bring these materials to each session. Do not give the caregiver more than one set of four cards after the first presentation of this lesson unless you are certain of the caregiver's and client's ability to work effectively with more material.
2. Instruct the caregiver to repeat the lesson each day at home.
3. Ask the caregiver to bring, in addition to the prepared materials, a list of grocery items in the home that he or she would like to have the client use in practice. Be certain to tell the caregiver not to practice with these items until they have been used in therapy.

Follow Up

1. This lesson should be repeated for a series of sessions.
2. If the client is able to work with additional sets of cards and if the caregiver agrees, add a second set or more, as required.
3. Before going on to Lesson Five, tell the caregiver and client that they are to pick out four items they plan to purchase at their next trip to the supermarket. Ask the caregiver to write these items on a blank sheet of paper and to bring it to the next session.

LESSON FIVE: USING THE SHOPPING LIST

Description of the Lesson

The client, with the aid of the caregiver, matches printed labels and pictures with simulated grocery items.

Goal

To enable the client to participate actively in the daily routine of running a household by assisting in shopping.

Objectives

- To improve list generation skills
- To improve naming skills
- To enhance memory
- To enhance writing skills

Materials

- Basket or box for grocery items
- Four simulated grocery items
- Matching set of picture labels
- Matching printed labels
- Blank cards for pictures and labels

Preparation

If the client and caregiver have completed Lesson Four, choose grocery items from the list generated at that lesson. If the client and caregiver have not completed Lesson Four, prepare a short list for use during this lesson.

COMMENTS	INSTRUCTIONS

Preliminary

Reality Orientation

The client is oriented to person, place, and time.

1. Greet the client and caregiver by name and show them into the therapy room. Example: "Good morning, Mrs. S. I'm Jane Doe, the (your title). It's nice to see you and Mr. S. Let's go into the therapy room."

·Instructions are concrete and offer no choices.

2. Upon entering the therapy room, instruct the caregiver and client to be seated together opposite you or to your left; therapy materials should be on a table near you but in clear view and within easy reach of everyone.

Step A

Tasks

1. Introduce the lesson. Example: "We are going to practice using a shopping list."

2. If Lesson Four was done, ask the caregiver for the client's shopping list and check the items on that list against the prepared materials.

3. If the client did not do Lesson Four, place the prepared list (now the client's list) before the client and caregiver and say, "We will use this as our shopping list."

COMMENTS	INSTRUCTIONS
	4. Ask the client to read one item from the shopping list. Example: "Mrs. S, read one item from the shopping list." If the client is unable to respond correctly, cue. Example: Point to the first word on the list and say, "This is something you drink." The caregiver should be encouraged to cue the client. If the client is unable to respond or circumlocutes, give the correct answer.

Step B

Tasks

1. Show the client a picture of the item and say, "This is a _____. What is this?"

2. Place the picture on a blank card.

3. Show the client the matching printed label and ask him or her to read it. If the client is incorrect or circumlocutes, give the correct response. If there is no response, cue.

4. Place the printed word beneath the picture on the card. Pointing first to the picture, then to the word, identify the item and ask the client to repeat.

Step C

Tasks

1. Place the simulated grocery items on the table for the client to see.

2. Place one card on the table before the client. Ask the client to find the matching grocery item.

COMMENTS	INSTRUCTIONS
	$\leftarrow$ 3. If correct, remove the item and the card and repeat from Task 1 until all items are matched.
	4. If incorrect, ask the caregiver to give the client the item.
	5. Point to the item and say its name. Ask the client to repeat. Point to the word, say it, and ask the client to repeat. Point to the picture, say the item's name, and ask the client to repeat.
	6. Remove the item and the card and repeat from Task 2 until all items are matched.

Activity Break

Compliment the client and caregiver on their teamwork. Commend the client on the effort put forth. Inform the client and caregiver that the exercise is almost complete.

Step D

Tasks

1. Place the grocery items back on the table before the client.

2. Give the caregiver the cards.

3. Give the client the basket or box.

Be certain to tell the caregiver that he or she is not to give the client a card at the supermarket until they are in front of the item to be purchased.

4. To the caregiver, say, "We are going to pretend that you are at the store. I want you to give Mrs. S. one card and ask her to find the item on the table."

5. If correct, have the client place the item in the basket and repeat until all items are in the basket.

COMMENTS	INSTRUCTIONS
	6. If incorrect, have the caregiver hand the client the item and name it.
	7. Have the client put the item in the basket.
	8. If the client cannot put the item in the basket, have the caregiver do so.
	Activity Break
	When all the items are in the basket, compliment the client and caregiver on their teamwork and tell them that they are to try matching picture-word cards to items on the shelf the next time they are at the supermarket.

Caregiver's Instructions

1. Give the caregiver four practice cards.
2. Instruct the caregiver to use the cards on the next trip to the supermarket in the following manner.

   a. The caregiver stops in front of the item to be purchased and hands the card to the client. The client is asked to find the item. The caregiver takes the item from the shelf, names it, and hands it to the client to put in the shopping basket.
   b. For items without cards, the caregiver finds the item, takes it from the shelf, names it, and hands it to the client to put into the basket.

3. If the caregiver discovers that the client can manage more than four cards in a single shopping trip, he or she should be encouraged to work with the client and make up additional cards.

LESSON SIX: UNPACKING THE GROCERIES

Description of the Lesson

Although the client in stage 2 of Alzheimer's disease cannot function without the aid of the caregiver, it is important to keep the client involved in meaningful activities. In this lesson the client, with the aid of the caregiver, identifies simulated grocery items and matches them to pictures and printed labels.

Goal

To enable the client to participate actively in the daily routine of the household by assisting in unpacking purchased items.

Objectives

- To improve naming skills
- To improve content of communication by reducing irrelevant responses
- To improve word recognition
- To improve picture identification

Materials

- Bag or box containing four to six grocery items that are always stored in the same location (for example, in the refrigerator or on a shelf in the cupboard)
- List of items that are in the bag
- Cards with matching peel-off pictures
- Cards with matching peel-off printed words

Site Adaptations

If the lesson is to take place in the ADL room, set the bag or box of groceries on the table before the arrival of the client and caregiver. Place a written list of the items and matching labels (if they are to be used) and picture cards at your place.

If the lesson is to take place in the client's home, instruct the caregiver about how to adapt the kitchen in advance. The caregiver is to have the bag or box of groceries on the kitchen table ready for your arrival. You and the caregiver should agree on the contents of the bag in advance. Ask the caregiver to leave room on the table for the list of grocery items, matching labels (if they are to be used), and picture cards. If the caregiver does not have labels and pictures, bring these materials.

If the client is able to tolerate a complex exercise, Lessons Six and Seven may be combined with or without the printed cards.

COMMENTS	INSTRUCTIONS

Preliminary

Reality Orientation

The client is oriented to person, place, and time.	1. Greet the client and caregiver by name. Example: "Good morning, Mrs. S. I'm Jane Doe, the (your title). It's nice to see you and Mr. S. Welcome to our activities room" (or, "I'm happy to be at your house").
The information presented is simple and concrete. Time is allowed between your comments for the client to respond.	2. Identify the exact location of the action and the action itself. Example: "We will work in the kitchen. We will unpack groceries."
Include the caregiver in the remarks.	3. Specify the purpose of the action. Example: "This practice will help you and Mr. S. remember what is in your cupboards."
	4. Instruct the client and caregiver to be seated at the table to your left.

Step A

Tasks

Instructions are concrete and to the point.	1. Describe the action as you begin. Example: Place four pictures (or fewer) before the client and say, "We are going to name these pictures."
Using the client's name will help to bring him or her to attention and direct the action.	2. Point to one picture and ask, "Mrs. S., what is this?" If the client is unable to respond or responds incorrectly, go to Task 4.
	3. Repeat until all pictures are named.
	4. Point to one picture and say, "This is a _____. What is this?"

COMMENTS	INSTRUCTIONS
	5. If the client is unable to respond or responds incorrectly, supply the correct answer then ask the client to repeat.
	6. Repeat Tasks 4 and 5 for each incorrect response.

Activity Break

Compliment the client on his or her efforts.

Step B

Tasks

1. Ask the caregiver to take one item out of the bag and to name it.

2. Ask the caregiver to show the item to the client and to repeat the name. Example: "Very good, Mr. S. Now show the _____ to Mrs. S. and tell her what it is."

3. Ask the client to repeat the item's name.

4. Ask the caregiver to give the item to the client.

5. Ask the client to place the item on the matching picture. Example: Point to the pictures and say, "Mrs. S., put this _____ on the picture of _____."

6. If correct, repeat from Task 1 until all four items are matched.

7. If incorrect, pick up the item, show it to the client, and name it.

8. Hold the picture next to the item and name the picture.

COMMENTS	INSTRUCTIONS
	9. Place the picture on the table before the client and then place the item on top of the picture.
	10. Point to the item and the picture and name both.
	11. Point and ask the client to name the item first, then the picture.
	12. Repeat Tasks 7 through 11 until all items are matched.

13. If the client is able to read single words, go to Step C after the *Activity Break.*

Activity Break

If the client is no longer reading single words, the lesson ends here.

Step C

Tasks

1. Show one printed card to the client and read the word on the card.

2. Ask the client to repeat the name of the item.

3. Ask the caregiver to point to the item.

4. Ask the client to put the card on the matching item. Example: Point to the item and say, "Put this _____ on the _____."

5. If correct, repeat from Task 1 until all items are matched.

COMMENTS	INSTRUCTIONS
Tasks 6 through 10 are to be done only when an incorrect response is given. Start with Task 1 for each item and continue until all items are matched.	6. If incorrect, pick up the item, show it to the client, and name it.
	7. Hold the card next to the item and read the word.
	8. Place the card on the table before the client and then place the item on top of the card.
	9. Point to the item and name it; point to the card and read it.
	10. Point and ask the client first to name the item and then to read the card.

Caregiver's Instructions

1. Return the practice cards to the caregiver.
2. Instruct the caregiver to repeat the lesson once a day using the same items.
3. If possible, the caregiver should select items that are used daily and are located near each other (for example, bread, cheese, cold cuts, and butter can all be kept on one shelf in the refrigerator).
4. Stress the importance of having all materials set up in advance for subsequent sessions in the home.
5. The caregiver may want to try doing this lesson before the start of a meal. At the end of the exercise, the client and caregiver then eat the items used for practice.

LESSON SEVEN: PUTTING THE GROCERIES AWAY

Description of the Lesson

The client and the caregiver learn how to use external devices (labels and pictures) as assistive devices in remembering household items and their locations. This lesson may be carried out in either an ADL room or in the client's home.

Goal

To enable the client to participate actively in the daily routine of the household by assisting in putting purchased items in their proper places.

Objectives

- To improve naming skills
- To improve content of communication by reducing irrelevant responses
- To improve word recognition
- To improve picture identification

Materials

- Bag containing four to six grocery items that are always stored in the same location (for example, in the refrigerator or on a shelf in the cupboard)
- Cards with matching peel-off pictures
- Cards with matching peel-off printed words (used only if the client can read single words)
- List of items in the bag

Site Adaptations

If the lesson is to take place in the ADL room, set the bag of groceries on the counter close to where they are to be stored before the arrival of the client and the caregiver. Place the shopping list and matching labels (if they are to be used) and picture cards next to the bag of groceries.

If the lesson is to take place in the client's home, instruct the caregiver about how to adapt the kitchen in advance. The caregiver is to have the bag of groceries on the kitchen counter ready for your arrival. You and the caregiver should agree on the contents of the bag in advance. Ask the caregiver to make a list of the items in the bag and to leave room on the counter for the list, matching labels (if they are to be used), and pictures. If the caregiver does not have labels and pictures, bring these materials.

COMMENTS	INSTRUCTIONS

Preliminary

Reality Orientation

The client is oriented to person, place, and time.

1. Greet the client and caregiver by name. Example: "Good morning, Mrs. S. I'm Jane Doe, the (your title). It's nice to see you and Mr. S. Welcome to our activities room" (or, "I'm happy to be at your house").

The information presented is simple and concrete. Time is allowed between your comments for the client to respond.

2. Identify the exact location of the action and the action itself. Example: "We will work in the kitchen. We will put some groceries away."

Include the caregiver in the remarks.

3. Specify the purpose of the action. Example: "This will help you and Mr. S. remember where your groceries are stored."

4. Explain that everyone will have to stand and do a little walking for this lesson.

5. Instruct the client and caregiver to join you at the counter. Materials are arranged before you, and the client and caregiver are to your left.

Step A

Tasks

1. Describe the action as you begin. Example: Take one item from the bag and place it before the client. To the client say, "We are going to put the groceries in this bag away."

Step A is used to demonstrate the caregiver's actions described in Step B. Instructions must be concrete and to the point.

2. Point to the item and ask, "Mrs. S., what is this?"

Using the client's name will help to bring him or her to attention and direct the action.

COMMENTS	INSTRUCTIONS
	3. If the client is unable to respond or responds incorrectly, supply the correct answer and then ask the client to repeat.
	4. If correct, praise the client and say, "Good, this is _____. We are going to put this _____ in the cupboard."
	5. Instruct the client and caregiver to follow you to the cupboard. Hand the client the item, touch a space on the shelf, and say, "Put the _____ here."
	6. Show the client the picture of the item and ask him or her to name it.
	7. Point to the picture and say, "This is _____." Point to the item on the shelf and say "This is _____."
	8. Peel the picture off the card and ask the client to place it on the shelf next to or under the item where it can be seen.
	9. If the client is unable to respond or responds incorrectly, demonstrate.
If the client cannot read single words, do not do Tasks 10 through 13.	10. If the client can read single words, show him or her the matching word card. Ask the client to read the word aloud.
	11. Point to the item on the shelf and say, "This is _____." Point to the picture and say, "This is a picture of _____."
	12. Peel the word off the card and tell the client to place it next to or below the picture so that both the picture and the word are easily seen.
	13. If incorrect, demonstrate.

COMMENTS	INSTRUCTIONS

14. Compliment the client and then say, "Now let's have Mr. S. help with the next one."

Step B

Tasks

In Step B the caregiver, guided by you, repeats the actions carried out in Step A.

1. Instruct the client and caregiver to return to the counter.

2. Ask the caregiver to take one item out of the bag and to name it.

3. Ask the caregiver to show the item to the client and to repeat its name. Example: "Very good, Mr. S. Now show the _____ to Mrs. S. and tell her what it is."

4. Ask the client to repeat the name of the item.

5. Instruct the client and caregiver to return to the cupboard. Ask the caregiver to hand the item to the client.

6. Ask the caregiver to touch a space on the shelf and to say to the client, "Put the _____ here."

7. Give the caregiver the picture card and instruct him or her to ask the client to identify the picture.

8. If incorrect, have the caregiver give the correct response and the client repeat.

9. Ask the caregiver to remove the picture and have the client place the picture on the shelf near or below the item.

COMMENTS	INSTRUCTIONS
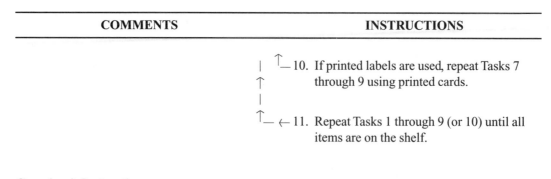	10. If printed labels are used, repeat Tasks 7 through 9 using printed cards. 11. Repeat Tasks 1 through 9 (or 10) until all items are on the shelf.

Caregiver's Instructions

1. Return the practice cards to the caregiver.
2. Instruct the caregiver to repeat the lesson once a day using the same items.
3. If possible, the caregiver should select items that are used daily and are located near each other (for example, bread, cheese, cold cuts, and butter can all be kept on one shelf in the refrigerator).
4. Stress the importance of having all materials set up in advance for subsequent lessons in the home.

LEVEL III

Functional Ability

As the disease worsens and cognitive abilities decrease, Alzheimer's clients may become severely disoriented. They may become confused as to who is a spouse and who is a parent or whether a room is the bathroom or the closet. At this stage, clients have difficulty with dressing and other ADLs. They cannot bathe alone, have difficulty with toileting, and may be incontinent. They may not be able to follow through on an action such as picking up a spoonful of food and putting it into the mouth.

Psychotic symptoms such as delusions, hallucinations, paranoid ideation, and severe agitation may become manifest. These symptoms may be an extension of the cognitive deficit as opposed to those of a true psychosis (Schneck, Reisberg, & Ferris, 1982). The therapist may note the following symptoms.

Speech and language:	The client's ability to communicate is severely impaired. Upon testing, there may be
	• minimal repetition
	• severely impaired comprehension
	• impaired pragmatics
	• tendency to lapse into an unintelligible mumble
Cognitive tasks:	Progressive loss of mental abilities, extremely poor performance on new tasks, and severely limited ability to process information.
Orientation:	The client is easily confused even in familiar surroundings; he or she appears to be unaware of surroundings, the year, the season, and so forth.
Number concepts:	Erratic.
Memory:	Very poor. The client is largely unaware of all recent events and experiences but usually retains some knowledge of his or her past. The client may forget the spouse's name but can distinguish between strangers and people who are familiar. The client can almost always recall his or her own name.
Additional observations:	The client
	• needs help starting a task
	• is unable to complete a task
	• has mild to moderate physical problems
	• has eating problems
	• has flattened affect

LESSON ONE: ORIENTATION TO PERSON

Description of the Lesson

In this lesson the client, with the assistance of the caregiver, identifies himself or herself and at least one significant other by name.

Note

A comfortable, calm atmosphere is important to the success of this lesson.

Goal

To help the confused client remain oriented to self and one or two significant others.

Objectives

- To increase verbal output
- To improve recognition skills
- To improve eye contact

Materials

- Picture of client
- Picture of one or two significant others (maximum, two)
- Picture of client with significant other (if available)
- Blank labels
- Lapboard or picture holder (if not seated at a table)
- Picture pocket (if seated at a table)

COMMENTS	INSTRUCTIONS

Preliminary

Establish eye contact with the client before proceeding. This can be done by saying the client's name or taking the client's hand.	1. Greet the client by name. Once eye contact is established, gesture to and identify yourself. Example: "Hello, Mrs. S. (Pause.) I'm (gesture) Jane, (pause) your _____ therapist."
Instructions are concrete and offer no choices.	2. Describe the activity. Example: Show the client pictures and say, "We are going to look at some pictures."
	3. The client and caregiver are instructed to be seated where everyone can see the therapy materials.

Step A

Tasks

Allow time for the client to respond, and be aware that responses will not be immediate. Proceed at a slow pace.	1. Show the client his or her picture. Ask the client to identify the picture.
	2. If the client does not respond, hand the client the picture and repeat the question.
	3. If correct after Task 1 or 2, praise the client and give the picture to the caregiver.
	4. If the client does not respond to either Task 1 or Task 2, point to the picture and ask the caregiver to identify it.
	5. Ask the client to repeat the name.
	6. Ask the caregiver to comment on the picture. Example: "When did Mrs. S. take this picture?"

COMMENTS	INSTRUCTIONS
	7. Point to the picture and ask the client yes or no questions. Example: "Mrs. S., do you like this picture?"

Activity Break

Compliment the client for his or her effort.
Place the picture in the picture pocket or holder.

Step B

Tasks

COMMENTS	INSTRUCTIONS
If the client is unable to do more than one task at a time, do not proceed to Step B or C. Repeat Step A using the same materials.	1. Introduce the new task. Address the client by name to gain eye contact.
	2. Say, "We will now look at a picture of someone else."
Do not accept an incorrect response without correcting.	3. Repeat Step A using a picture of a significant other. If the client's speech is irrelevant or incoherent, correct the response.

Activity Break

Place the picture used in Step B next to the picture used in Step A.

Step C

Tasks

COMMENTS	INSTRUCTIONS
In Step C the emphasis shifts from identification of individuals to identification of an action.	1. Introduce the new task. Address the client by name to gain eye contact.
	2. Say, "We will look at one more picture."
	3. Show the client the picture of himself or herself with a significant other.

COMMENTS	INSTRUCTIONS
	4. Ask the client to identify the picture. Example: "Mrs. S., what is happening?" and "Who is this?" Point to one person.
	5. If correct, praise the client. Give the picture to the caregiver. Skip to Task 9.
	6. If the client does not respond, hand him or her the picture and repeat the question.
	7. If the client does not respond, point to the picture and ask the caregiver to identify the activity.
	8. Repeat the caregiver's statement, then ask the client to repeat the statement. Give the picture to the caregiver.
	9. Ask the caregiver to comment on the picture. Example: "When did Mrs. S. take this picture?"
	10. Point to the picture and ask the client yes or no questions. Example: "Mrs. S., do you like this picture?"

Activity Break

Compliment the client for his or her effort. Place the picture in the picture pocket or holder next to the others.

Step D

Tasks

1. Show the client all three pictures. Touch each one and make a short statement about them. Example: "This is Mr. S. Mr. S. is your husband."

COMMENTS	INSTRUCTIONS
	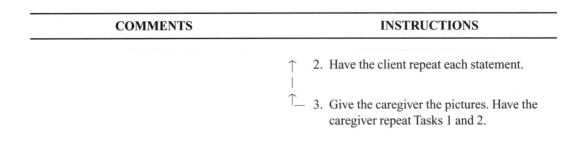 2. Have the client repeat each statement.

3. Give the caregiver the pictures. Have the caregiver repeat Tasks 1 and 2. |

Caregiver's Instructions

1. Instruct the caregiver to use the same pictures each time the lesson is repeated.
2. Instruct the caregiver to repeat the lesson in the same manner two times each day.
3. The caregiver should encourage as much talking as possible but not allow the client to ramble.
4. The caregiver should correct incorrect responses gently but firmly and have the client repeat correct responses.
5. The caregiver should allow time for the client to respond.
6. Eye contact is a must. To gain eye contact, the caregiver should address the client by name and touch the client's arm or shoulder.
7. The caregiver should reassure the client and praise all positive behaviors.

LESSON TWO: ORIENTATION TO PLACE

Description of the Lesson

In this lesson the client, with the assistance of the caregiver, identifies his or her immediate surroundings.

Note

This lesson is intended for home or institutional use. It will not be meaningful or useful for the client to practice this lesson in temporary surroundings.

Goal

To help the client remain oriented to place.

Objectives

- To increase verbal output
- To improve recognition
- To improve eye contact
- To improve object identification skills

Materials

- Brightly colored blank peel-off labels
- Marking pen

COMMENTS	INSTRUCTIONS

Preliminary

Establish eye contact with the client before proceeding. This can be done by saying the client's name or taking the client's hand.	1. Greet the client by name. Once eye contact is established, gesture to and identify yourself and the location. Example: "Hello, Mrs. S. (Pause.) I'm (gesture) Jane, (pause) your _____ therapist. I'm happy to be in your _____ room."
Instructions are direct and simple.	2. Describe the activity. Example: "We are going to look at things in your room."
If the client is ambulatory, guide him or her around the room and touch objects. If the client is not ambulatory, bring the objects to the client to touch.	3. The client and caregiver need not be seated for this lesson.

Step A

Tasks

Allow time for the client to respond, and be aware that responses will not be immediate. Proceed at a slow pace.	1. Show the client one object in the room. Have the client touch it and identify it.
	2. If the client does not respond, cue by saying "This is your room and this is your _____."
	3. If the client does not respond, ask the caregiver to identify the object.
	4. Ask the client to repeat the name of the object.
	5. Praise the client for each correct response.
	6. Ask the caregiver to print the name of the object on a label.

COMMENTS	INSTRUCTIONS

7. Peel off the label and assist the client in putting it on the object.

8. Point to the object and label. Have the caregiver identify them and the client repeat.

Activity Break

Compliment the client for his or her effort.

Step B

Tasks

Step B is the same as Step A except that it is carried out with a different object and a different color label. If the client is unable to change sets, skip Steps B and C.

1. Introduce the new tasks. Address the client by name to gain eye contact.

2. Say, "We will now look at something else in your room."

Do not accept an incorrect response without correcting.

3. Repeat the tasks in Step A with the second object and a different color label.

Step C

Tasks

1. Introduce the new tasks. Address the client by name to gain eye contact.

2. Say, "We will look at one more object."

3. Repeat tasks in Steps A and B with a different object and a different color label.

4. Tell the client the names of each object and have the client repeat.

5. Have the client use or handle the objects.

COMMENTS	INSTRUCTIONS
	6. Guide the client and caregiver around the room, identifying objects and having the client repeat each name.
	7. When the objects in the room have been identified, say to the client, "This is your room. These are your things." Have the client repeat the name of each object identified.

Caregiver's Instructions

1. Instruct the caregiver to be consistent and to repeat the lesson in the same manner two times each day, pointing to the labels.
2. The caregiver should encourage as much talking as possible but not allow the client to ramble.
3. The caregiver should correct incorrect responses gently but firmly and have the client repeat the correct responses.
4. The caregiver should allow time for the client to respond.
5. Eye contact is a must. To gain eye contact, the caregiver should address the client by name and touch the client's arm or shoulder.
6. The caregiver should reassure the client and praise all positive behaviors.

LEVEL IV

Functional Ability

In the last stage of Alzheimer's disease, the client no longer attempts to communicate with others. Physical and cognitive changes are severe, and the client, no longer ambulatory, appears to be unable to eat.

The therapist may note the following symptoms.

Speech and language: Speech is limited to a few words, and there is no intelligible vocabulary.

Additional observations:
- Loss of motor abilities
- Regression to fetal stage

As much contact as possible should be maintained with the client through touch, music, and direct speech. Formal communication therapy, however, is not suggested for clients in this stage.

Working with Dementia Clients in Long-Term Care Settings

RATIONALE FOR PROGRAM DEVELOPMENT

In today's health care market the term "long-term care" may have several different meanings. The most common meaning is "nursing home." In truth, "long-term care" covers a variety of permanent or semipermanent types of placements other than the person's home, and requires 24-hour paid staff. This includes personal care homes, facilities developed specifically to care for persons with dementia, and nursing facilities that have a continuum of skilled and unskilled levels of care. The common thread to all of these facilities is that they are institutional in nature and must adhere to a varying degree of regulations regarding staffing and programming. The vast majority of these facilities tend to provide little, if any, formal rehabilitative programs for their dementia residents. This occurs for two reasons. First is the nature of the disease. Since the disease itself cannot be affected or stabilized by medical treatment, many believe physical, occupational, and/or speech therapy cannot help. Second is the attitude of many professionals who not only believe treatment is futile, but reimbursement is not available. Given these two propositions it is little wonder that so few dementia residents are ever seen on a regular basis in the rehabilitation department.

In response to the need for formal programs developed specifically for this type of clientele, Glickstein Neustadt Inc. (GNI), a Pittsburgh-based company that provides contracted physical, occupational, and speech-language services, developed the GNI Action Oriented Program for Persons with Cognitive Disabilities (AOPPCD). AOPPCD utilizes both traditional and nontraditional treatment methods to achieve outcomes that are based on the individual's functional abilities and needs. The program's structure is based on Medicare and OBRA law, making it reimbursable and attractive to long-term care facilities.

On December 22, 1987, The Omnibus Budget Reconciliation Act of 1987 (OBRA-87), Pub. L. 100-203, was enacted. OBRA-87 included extensive revisions to the Medicare and Medicaid statutory requirements for nursing facilities. The law requires long-term care facilities participating in the

Medicare and/or Medicaid programs to conduct comprehensive, accurate, standardized, and reproducible assessments of each resident's functional capacity using a resident assessment instrument (RAI). The RAI is composed of the minimum data set (MDS), resident assessment protocols (RAPs), and triggers. The MDS is a minimum set of screening and assessment elements that must be used to assess an individual nursing home resident. The items in the MDS standardize communication within facilities, between facilities, and between facilities and outside agencies regarding resident problems and conditions. The facility *must* reexamine each resident no less than once every three months. The MDS is to be conducted by or under the supervision of a registered nurse with input from appropriate disciplines.

The current RAI contains 18 RAPs areas (Exhibit 9–1). The RAPs are structured frameworks for organizing MDS elements, as well as other clinically relevant information about an individual that contribute to care planning. Specific RAPs are used only when they are "triggered." A trigger is a specific resident response for one or a combination of MDS elements. Triggers identify residents who require further evaluation and/or management using the appropriate RAP(s). Since the MDS requires multidisciplinary input, as well as appropriate action to help the resident attain and maintain optimal function, the need for rehabilitative intervention in persons with dementia becomes obvious. Although residents in a Medicare certified "swing-bed" hospital, noncertified units of long-term care facilities, or licensed only facilities are not required by federal law to be assessed using the RAI, state law may require that *all* long-term care residents must be assessed.

SERVICE NEEDS OF THE ALZHEIMER'S CLIENT

The nature and degree to which any Alzheimer's client will need health and rehabilitation services depends on the client's current status and premorbid condition. A client's premorbid condition may

Exhibit 9–1 Resident Assessment Protocols (RAPs)

1. Delirium
2. Cognitive Loss
3. Visual Function
4. Communication
5. ADL Functional/Rehabilitation Potential
6. Urinary Incontinence and Indwelling Catheter
7. Psychosocial Well-Being
8. Mood State
9. Behavioral Symptoms
10. Activities
11. Falls
12. Nutritional Status
13. Feeding Tubes
14. Dehydration/Fluid Maintenance
15. Dental Care
16. Pressure Ulcers
17. Psychotropic Drug Use
18. Physical Restraints

range anywhere from perfectly healthy (no services needed) to frail (in need of multiple services). Therefore, determining which services are strictly for the remediation of Alzheimer's disease and which are needed for a pre-existing condition can be complicated. Thus, a therapist may find that a client being treated for arthritis needs additional services because of the onset of Alzheimer's disease.

Not all Alzheimer's clients have premorbid conditions requiring medical or rehabilitative therapy. In the case of the relatively healthy Alzheimer's client, a speech pathologist may be called in as part of the evaluating team to determine whether speech or language therapy is needed. Because changes in communication are a hallmark in dementia and are frequently noted as an early symptom, ongoing evaluation of communication and language changes is a minimum requirement. Therapy need not—and should not—last forever, but identification of problems and the establishment of sound communication programs are crucial. Through each phase of the disease the speech pathologist helps improve the communication necessary for proper treatment.

In addition to changes in communication, there are changes in the client's ability to handle day-to-day tasks such as dressing, bathing, and eating with utensils. As the disease progresses, an occupational therapist is needed to devise new strategies for ADLs. Although this book does not specifically address the physical therapy needs of the client, the physical therapist is an important member of the team. Muscle strength, balance, and gait training are all needed to help keep the client active, safe, and functional for as long as possible.

THE GNI ACTION ORIENTED PROGRAM FOR PERSONS WITH COGNITIVE DISABILITIES

The GNI AOPPCD is a goal-oriented program that uses functional abilities as indicators of change. Development of the AOPPCD was a joint effort of the departments of speech/language pathology, occupational therapy, nursing, social service, and activities of the Baldwin Health Care Center in Pittsburgh, Pennsylvania. The purpose of the program is to maximize the functional abilities of residents of a nursing facility diagnosed as having dementia. The program emphasizes functional communication/socialization and increased awareness of the surrounding environment. The initial target population for the program was "confused" residents who seemed unable, or refused, to participate in the general activities of the facility and were at risk for isolation and loss of skills.

Implementation of the program requires the specialized skills of an occupational therapist, certified occupational therapy assistant, and speech/language pathologist. Once the program is implemented, responsibility for its ongoing success is passed to nursing and activities. It is the responsibility of social service to act as a liaison to the families and to bring to the staff's attention any feedback on the program. The charge to the staff was to identify residents who are potential candidates for the program, and to develop appropriate programs that could be subsumed into the general milieu of the facility.

Identifying Appropriate Candidates

Clients living in the community generally enter a rehabilitation program via one of two routes: a physician's recommendation at an acute care facility, or by referral, generally from a physician, on an outpatient basis. Home care, skilled nursing, and some outpatient services are frequently a continuation of service that was initiated but not completed at an acute care facility. In the long-term care facility, the client may be referred to the therapist by a physician, nurse, psychologist, nursing assistant, activities staff member, or by the family.

For a resident to be eligible for the AOPPCD program, the resident must have a documented diagnosis of dementia as well as demonstrated reduced participation in structured activities and/or socialization with other residents. On the Minimum Data Set (MDS) – Version 2.0, the resident must have the following scores.

Section C. Communication/Hearing Patterns - Exhibit 9–2
    Item #4 (making self understood)   0, 1, or 2
    Item #6 (ability to understand)   0, 1, or 2
Section G, Physical Functioning and Structural Problems - Exhibit 9–3
    Item #7 (task segmentation)   1

Once the screening criteria have been met, the resident's family is invited to discuss the program and any reimbursement issues. For reimbursement purposes, the therapist must obtain the physician's order before proceeding with any evaluation or treatment plan.

Evaluation

To be successful, therapists who plan to work with dementia clients must first come to terms with their own desires and goals for their clients. It is a given that the client will *not* get well and in all probability will not make great gains. However, in addition to demanding an assessment and development of a plan of care for each resident of a skilled nursing home, the law states that each resident of a long-term care facility has the right to function at the highest level feasible. Facilities *must* provide physical, occupational, and/or speech therapy to those residents needing these services. Embedded within these two sentences are two questions that the therapist must answer before rehabilitation can proceed under the Medicare/OBRA guidelines. The first is "Can this person function better or safer?" If the answer to this question is uncertain or yes, then the rehabilitation professional must evaluate the resident to determine the client's potential level of function. This is not the same as determining the resident's rehabilitation potential. The term "rehabilitation potential" carries with it the connotation of traditional therapy and the corollary "significant progress." "Potential level of function" in its simplest form means "can this resident do better than he or she is currently doing, either with assistance or independently?"

The second question is "Does this resident require the rehabilitation professional's particular expertise to function at his or her best (safest)?" If the answer to the second question is "yes, the rehabilitation professional's skills and/or knowledge are needed" then a program should be developed. Not every evaluation will result in the development of a program. However, every program should be preceded by an evaluation. The goal is to help the resident function better or safer. Keep in mind that we are addressing quality of life issues and the resident may never achieve significant progress in any of the traditional rehabilitation spheres.

Whenever possible, Alzheimer clients should be tested using standardized tests. The initial test acts as a baseline and can be used to monitor the progression of the disease as well as any positive or negative changes in function. In the event the individual is unable to be evaluated using standardized measures, *nonstandardized probes* are appropriate. For example, observing the person during their morning ADLs or during a meal to evaluate his or her range of motion, ability to identify items of clothing and use them appropriately, ability to communicate needs, and so on could be used. Skilled observation is reimbursable under the Medicare Guidelines (see Unit 11).

A good rule of thumb is to choose tests that reflect the information needed to determine an action plan. While a lengthy test battery may be necessary to determine the existence and extent of a particular disorder, in the long-term care setting extended testing is rarely necessary to determine the individual's strengths and weaknesses within a functional environment. Therefore, the therapist may wish to

Exhibit 9–2 Minimum Data Set (MDS)—Version 2.0, Communication/Hearing Patterns (Section C)

1.	HEARING	*(With hearing appliance, if used)* 0. *HEARS ADEQUATELY*—normal talk, TV, phone 1. *MINIMAL DIFFICULTY* when not in quiet setting 2. *HEARS IN SPECIAL SITUATIONS ONLY*—speaker has to adjust tonal quality and speak distinctly 3. *HIGHLY IMPAIRED*/absence of useful hearing	
2.	COMMUNI-CATION DEVICES/ TECH-NIQUES	*(Check all that apply during last 7 days)* Hearing aid, present and used	a.
		Hearing aid, present and not used regularly	b.
		Other receptive comm. techniques used (e.g., lip reading)	c.
		NONE OF ABOVE	d.
3.	MODES OF EXPRESSION	*(Check all used by resident to make needs known)*	
		Speech `a.` / Signs/gestures/sounds	d.
		Writing messages to express or clarify needs `b.` / Communication board	e.
		/ Other	f.
		American sign language or Braille `c.` / *NONE OF ABOVE*	g.
4.	MAKING SELF UNDER-STOOD	*(Expressing information content—however able)* 0. *UNDERSTOOD* 1. *USUALLY UNDERSTOOD*—difficulty finding words or finishing thoughts 2. *SOMETIMES UNDERSTOOD*—ability is limited to making concrete requests 3. *RARELY/NEVER UNDERSTOOD*	
5.	SPEECH CLARITY	*(Code for speech in the last 7 days)* 0. *CLEAR SPEECH*—distinct, intelligible words 1. *UNCLEAR SPEECH*—slurred, mumbled words 2. *NO SPEECH*—absence of spoken words	
6.	ABILITY TO UNDER-STAND OTHERS	*(Understanding verbal information content—however able)* 0. *UNDERSTANDS* 1. *USUALLY UNDERSTANDS*—may miss some part/intent of message 2. *SOMETIMES UNDERSTANDS*—responds adequately to simple, direct communication 3. *RARELY/NEVER UNDERSTANDS*	
7.	CHANGE IN COMMUNI-CATION/ HEARING	Resident's ability to express, understand, or hear information has changed as compared to status of **90 days ago** (or since last assessment if less than 90 days) 0. No change 1. Improved 2. Deteriorated	

consider choosing those sections of functional tests that best reflect the skills needed for the potential client to function within a given setting. For example, Exhibit 9–4 is a cognitive profile being developed by GNI for occupational therapists. The profile consists of 27 tasks divided into eight areas of cognition: attention, orientation, memory, problem solving, organization/planning, judgement/insight, abstract thinking/mental flexibility, and perception. It is scored on a 6-point scale, 0–5. The tasks are all relatively low level and nonthreatening, but are sufficiently complex to allow the therapist to identify areas of strength and weakness. The test need not be given in the therapy room. In fact, the resident's own room may be the preferred area since the resident may be more comfortable and better oriented in

Exhibit 9–3 Minimum Data Set (MDS)—Version 2.0, Physical Functioning and Structural Problems (Section G)

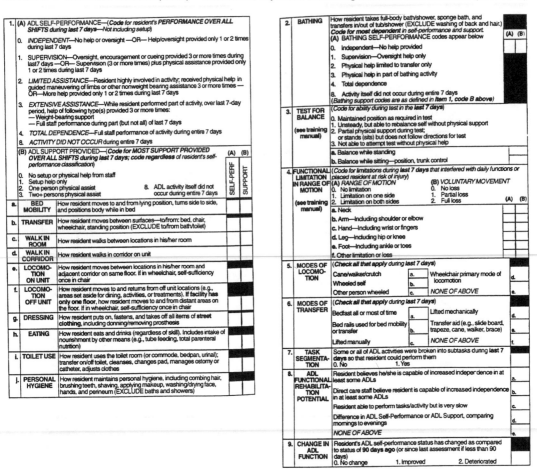

a more familiar environment. The reader should also note that some of the questions can be presented as part of a natural conversation. The resulting cognitive profile points to the resident's strengths as well as weaknesses, allowing the therapist to build on the strengths.

Regardless of how the potential client is evaluated, a consistent, ongoing, reproducible, task performance measure that can be used to document change in functional status once treatment has been terminated must be established. This measure need not be complex. For example, when working with residents who have difficulty during meals, it may be desirable to document how much of the meal is consumed (100%, 50%, or main dish and one side dish) or how long it takes the resident to eat (20 minutes independently, 15 minutes with assistance, etc.). By the time the formal rehabilitation program is terminated, a caregiver should have been trained to continue the restorative nursing program and know how to document the resident's task performance. Thus, the formal rehabilitation program becomes the restorative nursing program, resulting in continuity of care.

As stated earlier, not every resident will be a candidate for therapeutic intervention. Exhibit 9–5 is a dementia profile intended as a guide for identifying persons who might benefit from therapeutic interventions. In cases where the resident's medical condition is unstable, or where the disease process is too

Exhibit 9–4 GNI AOPPCD Cognitive Profile

Name _____   Date _____

Scoring

Responds to questions or tasks:

5. with no delays or errors
4. with delays and/or errors but self-corrects
3. with vague responses to questions; with cues/redirection is able to complete the task
2. does not know the correct response to question; unable to complete the task without assistance for structuring
1. response to question is unrelated to the question; unable to respond to structuring and redirection in tasks
0. no response to questions; unable to engage in tasks

	SCORE						
	5	4	3	2	1	0	
ATTENTION							1. Attends to task(s) for 15 minuutes.
							2. Attends to details.
ORIENTATION							3. Oriented to person.
							4. Oriented to place.
							5. Oriented to month and year.
MEMORY							6. Recalls 4/4 items shown after 2 minutes.
							7. Recalls 4/4 words.
							8. Recalls 4/4 words after 2 minutes.
							9. Gives accurate biographical information.
ORGANIZATION/ PLANNING							10. Sequences tasks.
							11. Sorts into 4 categories.
							12. Follows 3-step directions.
							13. Plans and executes multi-step process.
JUDGEMENT/ INSIGHT							14. Aware of own status/limitations.
							15. Interprets safety risks accurately.
PROBLEM SOLVING/ ABSTRACT THINKING							16. Able to make change involving 3 digits.
							17. Responds to 4/4 questions appropriately.
							18. Interprets proverbs.
							19. Shifts focus on task when needed.
PERCEPTION							20. Constructs clock with all components properly placed.
							21. Initiates donning a button-down shirt.
							22. Discriminates right and left.
							23. Names objects.
							24. Demonstrates gestures.
							25. Finds objects among other items.
							26. Identifies proper use of items.

continues

Exhibit 9–4 continued

Directions: Complete cognitive profile scoring sheet for the corresponding numbers ( ) in each of the following sections.

Section 1. Pose the following questions:

My name is _____. What is your name? (3)
Where are you from? (9)
What is your birth date? (9)
What is the name of this place? (4)
What brings you here? (14)

Section 2. Place a piece of paper and a book in front of the resident.
Ask the resident to open the book, place the piece of paper inside the book, then close the book. (12)

Section 3. Show the resident the card with 3 overlapping shapes and ask,
"Copy this design, then write today's date." (19) (5)
If the resident is unable to write the date, ask, "Can you tell me what today is?" (5)

Section 4. Show 4 items (comb, pencil, spool of thread, and paper clip).
Ask resident to name each item. (23)
Hand the resident one item at a time. Ask the resident: "Tell me what is this used for?" (26)
Then ask resident to: "Show me how you use this." (24)
Tell the resident you are going to cover the items and ask him/her to remember what they are.
Remove the items and set the timer for 2 minutes. When the timer goes off ask the resident to recall the items. (6)

Section 5. Show safety cards and ask what is wrong with each picture. (15)

Section 6. Pose the following four questions:

What would you do if you wanted to make a phone call and did not have money? (14)
What would you do if you received the wrong lunch tray? (14)
What would you do if you were having severe chest pain? (15)
What would you do if you wanted to attend an activity? (14)
Count the number of correct answers and score. (17)

Section 7. Tell the resident you are going to read a very brief grocery list. Say, "I want you to remember the items I name because I will ask you to repeat them." Read the list: bread, tomatoes, eggs, and cheese.
Ask the resident to repeat the list. (7)
Set the timer for 2 minutes and say, "That was very good. I will ask you to tell me the list again very soon."
When the timer goes off, ask the resident, "Remember the grocery list I asked you to repeat? I would like you to tell it to me again, now." (8)

Section 8. Ask the resident to draw a clock with the hands at 3 o'clock. (20)
If this task is correct, skip #9

Section 9. Ask resident to put the ADL sequence cards in order. (10)

Section 10. Place two boxes containing several items including a deck of cards in front of the resident.
Ask the resident to name the items in one box. (23)
Ask the resident to locate the playing cards in the box on the resident's left. (22) (25)

continues

Exhibit 9–4 continued

Ask the resident to sort the cards into suits. (11)

After ten cards have been sorted, ask the resident to sort the cards by numbers. (13) (19)

Section 11. Hand the resident the following items or pictures, one at a time, and instruct the resident

a) Stop sign— "Show me what this means." (24)

If the resident is unable to do this task, demonstrate and repeat your instructions then proceed to b) and c)

b) Tooth brush—"Show me how you use this."

c) Hammer— "Show me how you use this."

Section 12. Give the resident a shirt and instruct, "Show me how you put this on." (21) (10)

Section 13. Ask the resident, "What does _____ mean?"

A stitch in time saves nine. (18)

People who live in glass houses should never throw stones. (18)

Section 14. Ask the resident the following arithmetic problem:

If you had $2.00 and you bought something for $0.50 how much money would you have left?

(Answer $1.50) (16)

If the resident is not able to do this, present the money in change and repeat the question.

Section 15. Fill in the attention portion of the profile scoring sheet based on the resident's performance during the evaluation. (1) (2)

Source: Courtesy of GNI, Pittsburgh, Pennsylvania.

---

advanced, therapy is not recommended. The same is true for persons with uncontrolled violent or abusive behavior. By definition, any resident considered for a dementia program is permanently cognitively impaired and will, in all probability, have some combination of additional problem areas that need to be addressed.

Setting Goals and Objectives

Mager (1984) defines a goal as a general statement of what is to be accomplished. The goal tells where you want to be when you are finished doing whatever it is you are going to do. The objectives tell you what you need to be able to do along the way to the goal. You may need to accomplish several objectives before you reach your goal. For example, one goal in long-term care is to prevent or delay decline in the resident's functional status. Obviously, there is no single program or action that will accomplish this goal. However, when all of the departments involved in patient care work together to formulate an action plan, it may be possible to keep the resident physically and mentally functioning for a longer period of time than if he or she is left unchallenged or uncared for. For example, as a therapist you may find that a resident is able to dress if clothes are laid out properly, or eat safely when food is presented correctly, or walk without risk if a gait belt is used. By providing the appropriate program, the therapist interacts with the resident and the staff to prevent early decline and maintain the resident's current status. The therapist also helps to improve the client's quality of life by helping others to interact safely and appropriately with the client.

If the program is to be reimbursed, the therapist must request a physician's referral stating the reason for the referral. For example, "the resident is *at risk* for (falls, contracture, isolation due to decreased

Exhibit 9–5 Dementia Profile for Therapeutic Interventions

Intervention (Requires a diagnosis of Alzheimer's or related dementia by a physician and at least one or more of the following criteria.)	No Intervention (Person exhibits one or more of the following.)
1. Confused in any or all spheres (e.g., disoriented to person, place, or time).	Unstable medical condition.
2. Exhibits reduced inter/intra-personal skills (e.g., reduced socialization, withdrawal, depression).	Disease process is too advanced.
3. Exhibits memory and/or cognitive loss.	
4. Judgement and safety are impaired.	
5. Wanders, paces, or attempts to leave the facility/unit.	
6. Demonstrates odd/inappropriate behavior, hypo- or hyper-activity, personality changes, psychosocial changes.	
7. Difficulty with attention and concentration.	
8. Reduced awareness to limitations, others, environment.	
9. Demonstrates changes in communication (e.g., repetitive speech, stuttering, reduced responsiveness, loss in informational content during discourse, reduced comprehension, anomia) (Speech/language therapist).	
10. Requires min-max supervision and/or direction with any or all ADLs (e.g., feeding, bathing, hygiene, dressing, functional mobility/ambulation) (Occupational therapist).	Further modifications to the program are not required.
11. Gait instability or requiring assistance with mobility/ambulation (Physical therapist).	
12. Inability to locate their own room.	
13. Ability to identify concrete and/or abstract pictorial configurations.	
14. Difficulty with recognition of personal items, environment, people, objects.	
15. Difficulty associating objects with their related functions.	
16. Difficulty processing information and/or perceiving information heard.	
17. Incontinent of urine and/or stool but is able to be managed by one caregiver or moderated by schedule/behavioral stipulations.	
18. Difficulty with environmental cues, signs, distractions within the environment.	

continues

Exhibit 9–5 continued

19. Experiencing confusion as a result of change in the environment.	
20. Difficulty with sequential tasks during ADLs.	
21. Demonstrates acting out or abrasive behaviors (e.g., screaming, crying, calling out, table-hitting, unintentional hitting, or actual purposeful intent to harm others).	Exhibits excessive violent or abusive behavior.
22. Inability to imitate simple prompts.	
23. Difficulty with visual-spatial-perceptual relations.	
24. Not stimulable to therapeutic intervention or behavior modifications.	Does not benefit from therapeutic milieu.

Source: Courtesy of GNI, Pittsburgh, Pennsylvania.

communication, etc.)." Keep in mind, when a resident with Alzheimer's disease is not challenged to function at the highest level, he or she is at serious risk for losing those skills that are untapped.

If your goal is to keep a resident functioning at the highest level, you need to determine those objectives that must be reached in order to accomplish the goal. Objectives can and should be written in terms of functional outcomes. For example, if your goal is to delay decline in the resident's ability to ambulate safely, your objective may be to train the nursing assistant to walk (ambulate) the resident safely from his or her room to the dining area for meals three times per day, using a gait belt. The speech/language pathologist may set a goal to maintain safe and adequate nutrition and hydration with the objectives of training staff and family members to identify safe diet consistencies, provide appropriate foods, and use proper techniques for initiating a safe swallow; occupational therapy may wish to maintain the resident's independence in grooming by training the nursing assistant to set up wash cloth, basin of water, and soap, and to cue the resident in their use. Note that thus far we have been talking about maintenance programs. Although the majority of programs that are appropriate for persons who have been long-term residents of nursing facilities are maintenance programs, therapists should not overlook the possibility of short-term traditional therapy programs that culminate with an appropriate Functional Maintenance Program for residents who are able to follow simple directions. Residents who go out of the facility and return, who are put on or taken off a drug regimen, and who show a change in functional status need to be evaluated, and goals need to be adjusted to meet the resident's needs as well as abilities.

Developing Individualized Programs

The AOPPCD utilizes the Functional Maintenance Therapy (FMT®) model developed by GNI (Glickstein, J.K. & Neustadt, G.K., 1995). While a complete discussion of this system is beyond the scope of this book it is important to note that FMT is a rehabilitation service delivery model based on the Tri-Model philosophy of rehabilitation for long-term care. The two major goals of FMT are to maximize client function and to demonstrate the skilled nature of the service being provided. FMT involves the interdisciplinary team in the ongoing care of the client and ensures the provision of the much sought after continuum of health care to those who need it most. Goals in the FMT system include client, professional, and caregiver considerations. Client oriented FMT goals include

- identifying functional abilities
- maximizing functional abilities
- deterring and/or retarding the loss of functional abilities over time

Professionally-orientated FMT goals are to

- provide rehabilitation professionals with a service delivery model
- formalize the consultation process
- provide rehabilitation professionals with documentation tools that demonstrate the nature and quality of care and are acceptable to third-party payers

The FMT service delivery model is formatted to formalize the consultation process by focusing on six interrelated elements or steps necessary for the provision of a continuum of care to the client in long-term care. FMT is composed of

- screening
- the initial evaluation
- functional maintenance programs (FMP®)
- training
- appropriate documentation with forms reflecting the skilled nature of the service, and
- continuous quality assessment and improvement measures

Functional Maintenance Programs

The FMP® is a listing of recommendations and instructions used by caregivers and/or clients to enhance the client's abilities as identified during the evaluation. The FMP® serves both as a focus for training and as a documentation tool. Although GNI utilizes several different types of FMPs®, this discussion is limited to those programs developed for persons who do not fit into traditional therapy programs and to program adjustments. These include

- FMP® I, used when the results of the initial evaluation indicate no ongoing treatment (NOT) is warranted
- FMP® III, used when a change in client function necessitates an adjustment to the FMP® I

After screening and the completion of the evaluation process, for those individuals who are not appropriate candidates for ongoing (traditional) therapy, the development of programs designed specifically for functional maintenance become the focus of the consultation service. Since the individual is entering the therapy program at the maintenance level, the specific GNI form is labeled as FMP® I (see Exhibit 9–6). The objective of the FMP® is to ensure the client the treatment needed based on functional ability. The program provides the rehabilitation professional with a reference for the various stages of decline and/or recovery during rehabilitation and serves as a framework to justify services to physicians, residents, families, and third-party payers. Since no program will maintain the client forever, the therapist needs some mechanism to modify or adjust a program when there is a change—positive or negative—in the client's performance. In the event that the specific program needs to be adjusted due to a change in caregiver, environmental change, or inability of the caregiver or resident to accurately follow the program, the therapist may need to adjust the program by retraining caregivers, etc. When this occurs, the therapist modifies the current program and again provides a list containing the modified (adjusted) recommendations and instructions. The adjusted program is identified by GNI as FMP® III (Program Adjustment) (Exhibit 9–7).

Exhibit 9–6 Functional Maintenance Program I (FMP® I) No Ongoing Treatment (NOT)

P.T. ☐   O.T. ☐   SLP ☐   DYSPHAGIA ☐

Resident _____   B.D. _____

Medical Diagnosis _____   Onset _____

Rehab. Diagnosis _____   Onset _____

Physician _____   Referral Date _____

Facility _____   Therapist _____

Initial Evaluation Date _____   FMP® Completion Date _____

Based on the results of the Initial Evaluation, it has been determined that _____ is not an appropriate candidate for an ongoing treatment program. In order to maximize identified functional abilities, Functional Maintenance Therapy was provided. The Functional Maintenance Therapy took _____ hours to develop and institute and includes the initial evaluation, the designing of an individualized Functional Maintenance Program (FMP®), the inservicing of staff, and the education/training of the individual and/or family caregivers. The FMP® will be monitored if required on an infrequent basis by the rehabilitation professional.

The following FMP® is a Caregiver Advisory Program and/or a Resident Stimulation Program. Please note that the FMP® is on the reverse side of this page.

continues

Exhibit 9–6 continued

P.T. ☐   O.T. ☐   SLP ☐   DYSPHAGIA ☐

Resident _____   Facility _____

Physician _____   Therapist _____

FMP I

Therapist Signature _____   Date _____

Physician Signature _____   Date _____

Source: Courtesy of GNI, Pittsburgh, Pennsylvania.

Exhibit 9–7 Functional Maintenance Program III (FMP® III) Program Adjustment

P.T. ☐   O.T. ☐   SLP ☐   DYSPHAGIA ☐

Resident _____   B.D. _____

Medical Diagnosis _____   Onset _____

Rehab. Diagnosis _____   Onset _____

Physician _____   Referral Date _____

Therapist _____   Re-eval. Date _____

Prior Date of Service: From _____   To _____

Last Evaluated on _____   FMP® Adj. Completed On _____

Because the previous FMP® designed for _____ was no longer effective, a re-evaluation and adjustment has been provided. It took _____ hours to develop this FMP® and includes the re-evaluation, the time spent in revising the individual Functional Maintenance Program, the inservicing of staff, and the education/training of the individual and/or family caregivers. The FMP® will be monitored if required on an infrequent basis by the therapist.

reason for revision:

_____

functional abilities at time of last FMP®:

_____

functional abilities at time of monitor:

_____

functional abilities after FMP® adjustment:

*see other side for FMP®

Source: Courtesy of GNI, Pittsburgh, Pennsylvania.

Training Caregivers as Part of the Program

Given the nature of Alzheimer's disease, it is not always feasible to train the dementia client in the use of a specific technique. Regardless of whether the client is trained or not, as part of the FMP® the therapist will always train caregivers in the appropriate techniques or methods needed to stimulate the client's abilities. Training is carried out in the client's natural setting, that is, during the performance of ADLs, meals, activities, etc. This is particularly appealing in the long-term care setting where nursing assistants seldom have "extra" time to attend formal therapy sessions. As part of the caregiver training, the recommendations and instructions are documented on a progress note (Exhibit 9–8) and are reviewed with both staff and family caregivers. This review may be one-on-one with a specific caregiver, or in a group setting such as a care plan meeting or special inservice. Training by the therapist, when appropriately documented, is a reimbursable Medicare service.

It is important to remember that a Functional Maintenance Program is one step in Functional Maintenance Therapy. While it is feasible to develop maintenance programs that are effective and reimbursable without using the FMT® system, using the six elements of FMT® as a guide in program development helps to ensure coverage in the event of a denial. For a complete discussion of FMT® and FMP®, see Glickstein and Neustadt (1995), *Reimbursable Geriatric Service Delivery*.

Exhibit 9–8 Functional Maintenance Therapy® Progress Notes

P.T. ☐   O.T. ☐   SLP ☐   DYSPHAGIA ☐

Resident _____   B.D. _____   Sex _____

Facility _____   Physician _____   Room _____

FMP® Types   I ☐   II ☐   III ☐   FMP® Style: Advice ☐   Stim. ☐

FMP® designed by _____   Completed _____

FMP® being carried out by _____

Date	

RECORD OF TREATMENT NUMBERS INDICATE UNITS OF TREATMENT	ONE UNIT (1) = 15 MINUTES CIRCLED NUMBERS INDICATE UNIT FOR EVALUATION

MONTH	1	2	3	4	5	6	7	8	9	10	11	12	13	14	15	16	17	18	19	20	21	22	23	24	25	26	27	28	29	30	31	TOTAL

continues

Exhibit 9–8 continued

P.T. ☐   O.T. ☐   SLP ☐   DYSPHAGIA ☐

Resident _____   B.D. _____   Sex _____

Facility _____   Physician _____   Room _____

Date	

Source: Courtesy of GNI, Pittsburgh, Pennsylvania.

Medicare/OBRA Guidelines

(The following information has been excerpted from the *Federal Register*.)

A comprehensive assessment on each resident must take place within 4 days of admission (this has been changed to between 4 and 14 days of admission), effective October 1, 1990. Must be done initially and periodically. Promptly after a significant change in the resident's physical or mental condition; and in no case less often than once every 12 months. The NF must examine each resident no less than once every 3 months, and as appropriate, revise the resident's assessment to assure the continued accuracy of the assessment. The results of the assessment are used to develop, review, and revise the resident's comprehensive plan of care. Assessments must coordinate State required pre-admissions screening to avoid duplicative testing and effort.

The assessment will be coordinated by an RN. Each individual who completes a portion of the assessment must sign and certify the accuracy of that portion of the assessment. Effective October 1, 90 the comprehensive assessment will be based on a uniform data set specified by the Secretary and use an instrument that is specified by the state. It must: Describe the resident's capability to perform daily life functions and significant impairments in functional capacity.

The comprehensive assessment must include at least the following information: medically defined conditions and prior medical history; medical status measurement; functional status; sensory and physical impairments; nutritional status and requirements; special treatment procedures; psycho-social status; discharge potential; dental condition; activities potential; rehabilitation potential; cognitive status; and drug therapy. We propose at §483. 10(b)(1) that the resident has the right to be informed of his or her rights and the rules of the facility upon admission, in the language that he or she understands.

In the Quality of Life requirement at §483.15 we proposed that the facility must ensure that residents receive care in a manner and in an environment that maintains or enhances their quality of life without

Source: OBRA-*Federal Register*-Thursday, Feb. 2, 1989, Part II Department of Health and Human Services Health Care Financing Administration 42 CFR Part 405 et al. Medicare and Medicaid; Requirements for Long Term Care Facilities; Final Rule with Request for Comments.

abridging the safety and rights of others by a) treating each resident with dignity and respect, and b) maintaining each resident's privacy.

After examining comments received on the proposed quality of life requirement and on the proposed resident rights requirement, we have chosen to recognize the proposed quality of life requirement to include those provisions that best reflect an individual's ability to influence, and be influenced by, his or her physical and social environments and to participate fully in these environments to the full extent of his or her functional abilities.

Part 483-Conditions of Participation and Requirements For Long Term Care Facilities §483.25 Level A requirement: Quality of care Each resident must receive the necessary nursing, medical and psychosocial services to attain and maintain the highest possible mental and physical functional status, as defined by the comprehensive assessment and plan of care.(a) Level B requirement: Activities of daily living. Based on the comprehensive assessment of the resident, the facility must ensure that-

(1) A resident's abilities in activities of daily living do not diminish unless circumstances of the individual's clinical condition demonstrate that diminution was unavoidable, This includes the resident's ability to- (i) bathe, dress, groom, (ii) transfer and ambulate, (iii) toilet, (iv) eat and (v) to use speech, language or other functional communication systems.

(2) A resident is given the appropriate treatment and services to maintain or improvise his or her abilities specified in paragraph (a)(1) of this section and

(3) A resident who is unable to carry out activities of daily living receives the necessary services to maintain good nutrition, grooming, and personal and oral hygiene

(b) Level B requirement: Vision and hearing. To ensure that residents receive proper treatment and assistive devices to maintain vision and hearing abilities. The facility must, if necessary, assist the resident-

(1) in making appointments

(2) by arranging for transportation to and from the office of a medical practitioner specializing in the treatment of vision and hearing impairment or the office of a professional specializing in the provision of vision or hearing assertive devices

(g) Level B requirement: Naso-gastric tubes. Based on the comprehensive assessment of a resident, the facility must ensure that-

(1) A resident who has been able to eat enough alone or with assistance is not fed by naso-gastric tube unless the resident's clinical condition demonstrates that use of a naso-gastric tube was unavoidable; and

(2) A resident who is fed by a naso-gastric or gastrostomy tube receives the appropriate treatment and services to prevent aspiration pneumonia, diarrhea, vomiting, dehydration, metabolic abnormalities, and nasal-pharyngeal ulcers and to restore, if possible, normal feeding function.

§483.45 Level A requirement: Specialized rehabilitation services A facility must provide or obtain rehabilitation services, such as physical therapy, speech-language pathology, and occupational therapy, to every resident it admits.(a) Level B requirement: Provision of services. If specialized rehabilitation services are required in the resident's comprehensive plan of care, the facility must(1) Provide the required services; or (2) Obtain the required services from an outside resource...Assistive devices has been redesignated as§483.35(g) in this final rule and provides that the facility must provide special eating equipment and utensils for residents who need them.

In paragraph (b), Comprehensive assessments, we are requiring that each assessment must be conducted or coordinated with the appropriate participation of health professionals and effective October 1, 90, by a registered nurse who conducts or coordinates the completion of the assessment. In paragraph (b), we are including dental condition, activities, rehabilitation potential, drug therapy, and cognitive status among the required elements of a comprehensive assessment.

In paragraph (d), Comprehensive care plans, we require that the comprehensive care plan be prepared by an interdisciplinary team which after October 1, 90 includes the resident, resident's family or legal representative, a physician, a registered nurse, and other staff in disciplines determined by the resident's needs.

In reference to NG tubes-paragraph (h) - requirement that clinical conditions demonstrates that use of a nasogastric tube was unavoidable

We are requiring that all residents whose comprehensive assessment indicates rehabilitation potential receive, and the facility provide or obtain, appropriate rehabilitative services.

The SNF and ICF review process for certification will be simplified by combining two reviews into one. Focus is on outcomes.

(3) A resident who is unable to carry out activities of daily living receives the necessary services to maintain good nutrition, grooming, and personal and oral hygiene

(b) Level B requirement: Vision and hearing. To ensure that residents receive proper treatment and assistive devices to maintain vision and hearing abilities, the facility must, if necessary, assist the resident -

(1) in making appointments

(2) by arranging for transportation to and from the office of a medical practitioner specializing in the treatment of vision or hearing impairment or the office of a professional specializing in the provision of vision or hearing assistive devices

(g) Level B requirement: Naso-gastric tubes. Based on the comprehensive assessment of a resident, the facility must ensure that-

(1) A resident who has been able to eat enough alone or with assistance is not fed by naso-gastric tube unless the resident's clinical condition demonstrates that use of a naso-gastric tube was unavoidable; and

(2) A resident who is fed by a naso-gastric or gastrostomy tube receives the appropriate treatment and services to prevent aspiration pneumonia, diarrhea, vomiting, dehydration, metabolic abnormalities, and nasal-pharyngeal ulcers and to restore, if possible, normal feeding function.

{483.45 Level A Requirement: Specialized rehabilitation services A facility must provide or obtain rehabilitation services, such as physical therapy, speech-language pathology, and occupational therapy, to every resident it admits. (a) Level B requirement: Provision of services. If specialized rehabilitation services are required in the resident's comprehensive plan of care, the facility must (1) Provide the required services; or (2) Obtain the required services from an outside resource... Assistive devices has been redesignated as {483.35(g) in this final rule and provides that the facility must provide special eating equipment and utensils for residents who need them.

In Paragraph (b) Comprehensive assessments, we are requiring that each assessment must be conducted or coordinated with the appropriate participation of health professionals, and effective October 1, 90, by a registered nurse who conducts or coordinates the completion of the assessment. In paragraph (b), we are including dental condition, activities, rehabilitation potential, drug therapy, and cognitive status among the required elements of a comprehensive assessment.

In paragraph (d), Comprehensive care plans, we require that the comprehensive care plan be prepared by an interdisciplinary team which after October 1, 90 includes the resident, resident's family or legal representative, a physician, a registered nurse, and other staff in disciplines determined by the resident's needs.

In reference to NG tubes- paragraph (h) - requirement that clinical conditions demonstrate that use of a nasogastric tube was unavoidable

We are requiring that all residents whose comprehensive assessment indicates rehabilitation potential receive, and the facility provides or obtain, appropriate rehabilitative services.

The SNF and ICF review process for certification will be simplified by combining two reviews into one. Focus is on outcomes.

(Subsequent guidelines have dropped the "level A" and "level B" designations and have placed all requirements on an equal footing. [Author's note.])

Documentation

While proper documentation is always important to good care, documentation takes on an added dimension for anyone working with Alzheimer's patients. Let us consider some of the reasons why documentation is a crucial element of care when working with dementia clients. First, since Alzheimer's disease is considered to be a "red flag" diagnosis, clinicians must be prepared for additional scrutiny of any claims made for reimbursement. It is because claims reviewers use documentation in making coverage decisions that the clinician needs proper documentation to optimize chances for reimbursement through third-party payment. Second, the clinician's clear documentation is needed by physicians in caring for their patients. This means that the clinician needs some orderly method of identifying goals, progress, and problems when working with the client. Third, and to some most importantly, documentation is required by law. Documentation serves as a legal record of what has been done and why. Federal and state reviewers use documentation in making licensing decisions. Judges use documentation in rendering legal decisions.

The adage "if it wasn't written, it wasn't done" applies to rehabilitation professionals who may not have a focus for their client management suggestions. Rehabilitation professionals are often asked to evaluate clients who are not candidates for ongoing treatment. Informal suggestions become formal recommendations and instructions only when they are written. Establishing suggestions as written recommendations and instructions is an important training tool for use with the client and staff and/or family caregivers. In addition, a written recommendation is tangible information for the caregiver of an outpatient or resident, or to submit during care conferences. Consider the following: Many clients entering nursing homes are at risk for losing latent and/or dormant functional abilities that are not stimulated. In such cases the caregivers and the client need information gained during the initial evaluation to promote the client's functional use of identified skills, and/or training in carrying out specific stimulation tasks. The skilled nature of this service is established through the documentation of recommendations and instructions. This action improves interdisciplinary team communication and serves to advocate on behalf of the client.

Exhibit 9–6 is an example of a maintenance discharge form used to instruct caregivers and to alert professionals to the fact that this client was not placed on a traditional therapy program. Note that the form lets the reader know that no ongoing treatment (NOT) is recommended. Instructions to the caregiver are listed on the back of the form. During the care conference, these recommendations can be incorporated into the client's care plan. This approach improves the rehabilitation professionals' communication with each other, with members of the interdisciplinary team, with nonprofessional staff caregivers, and with family caregivers, thus improving the quality of care provided.

USING A GOAL-ORIENTED APPROACH

In today's health care climate a goal-oriented approach to documentation that states behavioral objectives and functional outcomes is recommended. The focus should be the specific problems—speech and language functions, ADLs, and the like—and outcome expectancies. Describing the therapeutic objective in terms of behaviors that can be observed and measured helps to show successive steps in client progress toward a functional goal. Practical outcome expectancies such as "Mr. Smith will communicate his need to ___" should be emphasized rather than abstract goals, such as "improved communication."

The goal-oriented method is used in the lesson plans given in Unit 8. First, a general or long-range goal is stated. The long-range goal is followed by a list of objectives or short-term goals. For example, in Level I, Lesson One, the long-range goal is to enable the client to write a brief letter or note to a family member, relative, or close friend. The immediate objectives of the lesson divide the goal into smaller segments that can be addressed in specific tasks. The first objective listed is to improve writing skills. The therapist, when documenting, may expand this objective to read "To improve writing skills by having the client identify pictures of family members and write each person's name on a lined piece of paper." Some therapists may choose to document in greater detail, as shown in the following example.

> Objective: To improve writing skills
> Method:
>   (1) After the client has identified a picture of a family member, the client will write the individual's name.
>   (2) The client will verbally describe the action shown in the picture.
>   (3) The client will write the action described using short sentences.

Not all goals are therapy oriented, and the speech pathologist or occupational therapist who chooses to document as the prime goal "To maintain social contact" without any additional information may be denied reimbursement. Therefore, therapy goals and objectives should always be stated in terms of the therapist's job description and scope of practice. For example, "To maintain social contact by increasing meaningful verbal output" or "To train staff in appropriate communication techniques which will encourage Mrs. Smith to engage in social interaction" are more appropriate goals.

CRITERIA FOR PROPER DOCUMENTATION

In addition to letting others know what the therapist and client have been doing, good documentation fulfills the following criteria.

Establishment of a Baseline from Which Changes Can Be Measured

Many reported changes in client behavior appear to be both subjective and variable. It is important for the therapist to establish the current functional level of the client by means of both objective and subjective measures. Reporting the results of measures such as the BDAE (Goodglass & Kaplan, 1972) and the ADL Scale (Katz et al., 1963; Fortinsky et al., 1981) with information reported by a caregiver is one method of establishing a baseline that can be used in future evaluations. Once a baseline is established, the therapist must decide whether or not intervention is appropriate and offer a prognosis, not on the course of the disease but on whether or not the client's functional level can be significantly increased by therapy or impacted positively via a maintenance program.

Maintenance of a Historical Record (Progress Notes)

An accurate historical record allows the therapist to make comparisons among current procedures and to prepare new procedures. Information regarding previous sessions is also needed when determining the effectiveness of a given procedure. For example, at session 1 Mr. B. was unable to follow a one-step command. After three therapy sessions at which specific goal-oriented techniques were used, Mr. B. was responding correctly three out of four times to specific one-step commands. Here the therapist has demonstrated that the client has made progress.

When working with moderate to severe dementia clients it is more than likely that the client will not make progress in the traditional sense of the word. For these clients documentation indicates the progression of services provided to establish the maintenance program. When establishing a maintenance program the clinician must document all of the activities that are involved in the plan. This includes design time for a program, education and training of caregivers, as well as any skilled observation and/or hands-on treatment. Note that in establishing a maintenance program it is the caregiver rather than the client who is most likely being trained. It is sometimes useful to use a progress note such as the one in Exhibit 10–1 that identifies the program as a maintenance program. Since the maintenance program may be of very short duration, ten or twelve visits over a two- or three-week time period, the treatment dates and number of units are included on the progress note. Instead of a weekly progress note, the therapists writes a summary of what was done on the day it was done and indicates the amount of time, in units, at the bottom of the sheet.

Writing a Discharge Summary

When the program has been completed, the therapist must write a discharge summary. Discharge summaries for maintenance programs should include instructions to the caregiver(s). To be effective, the instructions must be written at an appropriate level for the caregiver. Writing for caregivers can be a formidable task, since the therapist must learn to translate all jargon into layman's terms. The appropriate place for the jargon or professional language is in the evaluation. When writing, keep in mind who will read your documentation. The purpose of the evaluation is to tell the physician and other professionals that a skilled professional has made an appraisal of the resident's condition, and based on the results of specific tests, has reached the stated conclusions. The discharge summary serves a somewhat different purpose. While the summary should let the professional know the status of the resident at the conclusion of the program, it must also provide information to others about continuing the program after the therapist withdraws. Terms and abbreviations such as "ambulate" or "ROM" should be avoided or the instructions may be ignored. Instead the writer needs to use words such as "walk" or "stretch." Avoid telling the caregiver to "verbally cue" the resident. Instead say, "Tell John to ____."

Demonstration of the Quality and Effectiveness of Care

A therapist may do an outstanding job with a particular client, but if nothing is written an outside party may conclude that no service was delivered. It is important for the therapist to document suffi-

Exhibit 10–1 Functional Maintenance Therapy Progress Notes

P.T. ☐   O.T ☐   SLP ☒   DYSPHAGIA ☐

Resident Jane D.   B.D. 4/19/24   Sex F

Facility ABC Nursing   Physician Dr. Goodheart   Room Room 241W

FMP® Types   I ☒   II ☐   III ☐   FMP Style: Advice ☐   Stim. ☐

FMP® designed by: Nancy Smith, MA, CCC   Completed 2/15/97

FMP® being carried out by: _____ CNA (Nursing Staff) _____

Date	
2/3/97	See evaluation
2/4/97	Spoke with resident's family regarding establishing a communication program.
	Requested the family bring in pictures of significant events in the resident's life so that we can develop dialogue triggers.
	Discussed the resident's communication needs with nursing and CNA. Staff would like to know what prompts to use when they want Mrs. S. to participate in her program.
	Observed Mrs. S. and staff. Noted significant delay in Mrs. S. response time (greater than 7 seconds).
	Developed FMP

RECORD OF TREATMENT
NUMBERS INDICATE UNITS
OF TREATMENT

ONE UNIT (1) = 15 MINUTES
CIRCLED NUMBERS INDICATE
UNIT FOR EVALUATION

MONTH	1	2	3	4	5	6	7	8	9	10	11	12	13	14	15	16	17	18	19	20	21	22	23	24	25	26	27	28	29	30	31	TOTAL
February			⑥	4	4	2	3			4		2		2	1	DC																28

continues

Exhibit 10–1 continued

P.T. ☐		O.T. ☐	SLP ☒	DYSPHAGIA ☐

Resident __Jane D._____   B.D. __4/19/24_____   Sex __F_____

Facility __ABC Nursing____   Physician __Dr. Goodheart_____   Room __Room 241W_____

Date	
2/5/97	Family brought in pictures of Mrs. S. as a young girl, her wedding and
	several other family events. Reviewed pictures with Mrs. S. She became
	very animated when shown her wedding picture and responded orally to
	questions. Following this dialogue, she was willing to go with me to the
	dining room for lunch.
	Dialogue was then started with CNA. Incorporated pictures into FMP.
2/6/97	Developed a series of picture prompts to be used by CNA
2/7/97	Trained CNA in use of picture prompts during activities. Discussed
	delayed response time.
2/10/97	Met with family. Trained family in use of picture prompts, emphasized
	latency of response. Adjusted visual materials to meet resident's need to
	communicate basic wants and feelings (hot, cold, happy, sad) using
	picture prompts
2/12/97	Observed CNA with resident. Reviewed FMP. Had CNA sign training
	contract for FMP
2/14/97	Incorporated FMP into care plan. Trained staff
2/15/97	Observed family with resident using FMP
2/16/97	DC

ciently that others can know what procedure was chosen, why it was chosen, what the outcome expectations and actual outcomes were, and what future plans have been made.

Demonstration of the Level of Care Needed for the Client to Achieve Stated Goals

The therapist, by making chart notes and other documentation, must let others know that the procedure being implemented requires professional skills. It is as important to document problems and the lack of progress as it is to document progress. This indicates that professional services are needed if the client is to succeed. Documentation is also needed to justify changes in the treatment plan. A therapist who gets carried away describing the wonderful progress the client has made but does not document problem areas may find services terminated by an evaluator who feels that the client no longer needs professional help.

Provision of Proper Information for Reimbursement Claims

With proper documentation, the client's insurance may reimburse for (1) evaluation as part of the diagnosis; (2) a short-term treatment program, providing that the client has a potential for improvement; (3) establishing a maintenance program; and (4) evaluation at periodic intervals. There are many gray areas in reimbursement that are open to interpretation by the claims reviewer. Documentation is the practitioner's way of letting the payer know that the service billed was valid, well done, and effective. When documenting, it is important to indicate that the client's performance rather than the disease is being affected.

HOW TO DOCUMENT

One of the most innovative changes in health care has been the introduction of the Problem Oriented Medical Record (POMR) (Lewis & Deigh, 1973). Designed by Lawrence Weed at the University of Vermont, the POMR was originally intended for medical record keeping purposes (Bouchard & Shane, 1977). Its logical format and simplicity make it easily adaptable to other disciplines. The problem-oriented method is based on (1) collection of data, (2) identification of problem areas, (3) formulation of a treatment plan, and (4) follow-up information.

Various formats for reporting data adapted from the POMR have been used by professionals. Many therapists have their own particular method of documentation based on what they are comfortable with and the policies of their workplace. Those who do not already have a method will find that problem-oriented or SOAP formats can be helpful approaches to documentation. The letters in the acronym SOAP are derived from the type of information to be used in the progress notes: subjective, objective, assessment, and plan.

The following hypothetical case history illustrates documentation by means of a problem-oriented and a SOAP format.

> Mr. B., aged 68 years and with a history of rheumatoid arthritis, was admitted to an acute care facility because of an arthritis flare-up. Although he had agreed to hospitalization, once admitted he became uncooperative and did not fully participate in his rehabilitation program. To complete his therapy program successfully, Mr. B. needed to follow the therapist's directions during therapy and be able to continue his exercises on discharge. The physical therapist noted that Mr. B. was experiencing communication difficulties that sometimes made him hostile. His responses, at times, appeared to be bizarre. In addition, Mr. B. had difficulty following directions. When left alone he would start his exercise and then stop before finishing.

Mr. B.'s behavior was charted, and the physician ordered a complete evaluation of his physical and mental status. Since the staff reported difficulty communicating with Mr. B., in addition to ordering a neuropsychological evaluation the physician also ordered a speech and language evaluation.

Problem-Oriented Format

The problem-oriented format is frequently divided into three or four segments.

1. Statement of the client's current abilities. This is the data collection section of the documentation forms. Current history and test results are placed in this section.
2. Statement of the problem areas. These should be listed numerically.
3. Treatment plan. Treatment should be based on problem identification and include some statement regarding future goals and any need for additional testing.
4. Prognosis. The therapist should offer information regarding outcome expectancy of treatment. Prognosis is sometimes included as part of the treatment plan.

Initial Documentation for the Speech Pathologist

1. Statement of the client's current communication abilities
   Although Mr. B.'s speech in a social situation was appropriate and to the point, word-finding difficulties and circumlocution were evident. Mr. B. apologized for his inability to perform specific tasks and remarked that he noticed a change in his abilities. He could no longer read "long things" or concentrate. He said that this made him feel "dumb" and "angry." Mr. B.'s wife was very supportive of her husband and noted that "some days are better than others." Mrs. B. stated that her husband frequently went to the store alone but would sometimes return with the wrong item or incorrect change. When confronted, Mr. B. would deny the occurrence.

   Comprehension of information
   Mr. B. appeared to be confused and had difficulty responding to yes or no questions from the BDAE. He requested several repetitions of each question and offered elaborated explanations of his answers. Mr. B. read aloud a short paragraph, but his reading comprehension was limited to single words and sentences. Concept formation was concrete, as evidenced by his difficulty interpreting proverbs. Mr. B. displayed 75% accuracy in body part recognition. He was successful in pointing to pictures and colors.

   Ability to follow directions
   Mr. B. is able to follow a two-step command. When presented with a three-step command, he performed the first two steps successfully and requested a repetition of the third step. Mr. B. performed best when visual cues accompanied verbal commands.

   Information retention and retrieval
   There was a delay in Mr. B.'s response time to all stimuli. He was able to recall three objects after a period of 3 minutes.

   Expressive abilities
   Syntax and prosody were sound. As the length of utterance increased, however, there was a noticeable increase in circumlocution, digression, and empty discourse. When asked to interpret the "cookie theft" picture from the BDAE, Mr. B. requested several repetitions before identifying several of the objects in the picture. He did not comprehend the incongruities in the picture. His writing skills were also affected. When assisted, Mr. B. completed a brief note to his son.

Physiological status with regard to communication
Results of a CT scan and neuropsychological examination indicated a loss in cognitive skills and probable dementia. There was no evidence of stroke or any other physiological conditions that might interfere with communication. Hearing and vision were corrected to within normal limits.

2. Statement of problem areas

   - Inability to follow complex commands as a result of reduced auditory comprehension
   - Reduced ability to comprehend written materials
   - Reduced writing skills
   - Reduced verbal and word-finding skills
   - Concrete concept formation
   - Easy distraction from a task
   - Set-changing difficulties

3. Goals and treatment plan

   - Increase client's ability to follow verbal directions
   - Increase client's ability to follow written directions

4. Prognosis
   At this time Mr. B. can be taught to use his residual communication skills more efficiently through a set pattern of communication responses and by manipulating the environment.

Initial Documentation for the Occupational Therapist

1. Statement of the client's current functional status
   ADLs (feeding, bathing, dressing, preparing meals independently or with assistance from others)
   Mr. B. eats finger food without difficulty. When presented with silverware, he attempted to cut his meat with a spoon. Mr. B. can dress himself with assistance with buttoning and tying [scores on tests such as the Physical Self-Maintenance Scale (Lawton & Brody, 1969) or the Modified Barthel Index (Fortinsky et al., 1981) should be included].

   Limitations in range of motion and strength
   Observation of Mr. B.'s performance indicated that his functional range of motion was within normal limits.

   Perceptual problems
   Mr. B. had an eye examination on (date) and was wearing prescription glasses. He scored 75% on tests requiring pointing to body parts on request, figure ground identification, and completing a jigsaw puzzle of a person.

   Affect, motivation, and ability to follow directions
   Mr. B. maintained a good affect and was very sociable. He was unable to follow complex commands but responded well when information was presented in single steps with both verbal and visual cues. He was highly motivated and attempted all tasks.

   Family or caregiver involvement
   Mr. B.'s wife appeared to be very supportive, and she expressed interest in helping her husband.

2. Statement of problem areas

- Difficulty with dressing
- Difficulty using utensils because of visual perceptual problems
- Difficulty following complex commands
- Short attention span

3. Goals and treatment plan

- Improve Mr. B.'s ability to perform ADLs by teaching him a set response to a series of simplified instructions combined with verbal, visual, and tactile cuing.

4. Prognosis

Mr. B.'s awareness, motivation, and aspiration are all favorable prognostic signs. At this time Mr. B. appears to respond positively to manipulation of the environment and task-oriented instructions.

Follow-up Documentation (Similar for Both Disciplines)

1. Restate goals.
2. State progress achieved toward goals. Provide documentation related to the status of the client at the time. Relate this information to the need for additional therapy and prognosis.
3. Report on progress in areas not on the goal list.
4. Summarize current problems. Provide documentation of any problems that may be influencing the rehabilitation process, such as a lack of motivation or change in medical status.
5. Propose new goals. Indicate what the expected outcome would be, the reason for addition of or change in goals, and the need for continued therapy.

SOAP

A second method of documentation that uses a problem-oriented record is the SOAP format. The meaning of the acronym is as follows.

S—**Subjective** information pertinent to the client's behavior that is relevant to therapy is placed in this section. It is acceptable here to use terms such as "seemed" or "appeared to be." This is the section where information gathered from family members appears.

Example: Mr. B. appeared to be frustrated by his inability to complete tasks. His wife reported that he was easily frustrated at home. Both Mr. B. and his wife seemed to be highly motivated to perform well.

O—**Objective** measures such as test results and changes in performance scores belong in this section.

Example: Mr. B. achieved 75% correct responses in identifying body parts. He was able to follow two-step commands but was confused when presented with more complex stimuli. He could not visually identify his razor or comb.

A—**Assessment** is made by analyzing the subjective and objective information. It is important to incorporate both positive and negative or problem areas into this section to let others know whether therapy should be continued or terminated. It is also important to include a prognosis.

Example: Information gathered from Mr. and Mrs. B. indicates that Mr. B.'s primary area of need is ADLs, particularly grooming. Testing indicates that Mr. B. is able to carry out specific tasks needed to improve grooming by following two-step commands. The therapy goal is to improve Mr. B.'s use of grooming objects (comb, razor, and so forth).

P—**Plan** for the next session and state how this plan relates to the overall goal. The final step is to incorporate the subjective, objective, and assessment information into the plan.

Example: Begin establishing a daily grooming routine. Using visual, verbal, and tactile cuing, Mr. B. will identify his electric razor and use it to shave.

Charting Practices

Regardless of what method the therapist uses to document, if the therapist does not observe good documenting habits there will be little chance for reimbursement. De Millano (1984) lists six charting practices for nurses that should be followed by anyone documenting information.

1. Expect your document to be read by others. If your handwriting is difficult to read, print.
2. Allow sufficient time at the end of each session to record. Do not put it off.
3. Write enough to let the reader know what was done and why, but get to the point quickly. Stay with the subject matter. Do not put in extraneous or irrelevant information.
4. Use all the lines and spaces provided. Either draw a line or write "not applicable" if you do not use a space.
5. Use only standard abbreviations. If in doubt, write it out.
6. Identify your work by signing your full name and title on every page. Remember, this is a formal document (p. 32).

DOCUMENTING A FUNCTIONAL MAINTENANCE PROGRAM

User-friendly Functional Maintenance Programs (FMP®s) are among the most difficult types of programs to document. The degree of difficulty appears to lie in the requirement for absolute simplicity and clarity of purpose. The language of the FMP® must be geared to the user, generally a layperson with little or no knowledge of the therapist's field and even less background in jargon. The FMP® forms developed by GNI are discharge forms whose intended use is to instruct and remind the caregiver as to the proper technique in carrying out the plan of action. The FMP® I form shown in Exhibit 9–6 is a documentation tool designed specifically for use with individuals who are not appropriate candidates for therapy. In the event the claim is questioned, the front of the form contains all of the information needed by a reviewer to know that this was a maintenance program. The obverse of the form contains the program that is to be carried out by the caregiver. The program is written as a series of recommendations and/or instructions to the caregiver. Note that the sentences are short and to the point. Jargon is reserved for the evaluation, where it is necessary for the therapist to show the skilled nature of the service.

FMP®s should be incorporated into the client's care plan during the care conference. The language used must be easily understood by all caregivers. The therapist identifies and prioritizes the resident's concerns, needs, and problems. Specific time-referenced goals and objectives are then delineated and the approach or action to be taken is outlined.

Although proper documentation will not guarantee third-party payment, it will go a long way toward showing that therapy has been within the guidelines set by the intermediary or carrier for reimbursable services. In addition, documentation helps in the therapy process by allowing the therapist to determine the effectiveness of a given procedure and to plan future procedures.

Reimbursement and Regulations

REIMBURSEMENT

Therapists considering treatment of Alzheimer's clients frequently ask, "Will my services be reimbursed by a third-party payer?" Many professionals and family members of Alzheimer's clients are under the erroneous impression that rehabilitation services to an Alzheimer's client are not reimbursed by third-party payers because the client is unable to make "significant" progress. While payment may not have been available when dementia was considered a normal part of the aging process, that is not the case today. Certainly, evaluations prescribed by a physician are reimbursable. So too is a short period of therapy when indicated and properly documented. Understanding the type of insurance coverage as well as the regulations governing that policy (including limitations), and maintaining good documentation are keys to coverage. The therapist's best bet is to find out what the client's policy covers and to follow those procedures that allow an outside reviewer to understand the reasons for, and the nature of, the services provided. Remember, Medicare is an insurance policy governed by federal regulations. Clients who do not qualify for Medicare coverage may have other types of insurance. If a claim is denied, the therapist should go through the appeals process. When properly documented, most Medicare claims receive positive outcomes following an appeal.

Whether or not any health-related service is covered by third-party payment depends on three factors:

1. the type of policy the client has (for example, some policies cover rehabilitation services only in an acute care setting or at a skilled nursing facility);
2. the specific wording of the policy regarding a particular treatment (for example, "treat to overcome effects of pathological problem;" "maintenance if prescribed by a physician"); and
3. the wording used when documenting a claim (the insurer needs to know that the therapist is delivering service within the specific guidelines stated by the policy).

Since commercial insurance benefits are so highly variable and subject to change, it is the therapist's responsibility to check with the client and the insurer regarding specific reimbursement policies.

Reimbursement Mechanisms

Reimbursement for health care services has been going through a major evaluation and adjustment in service coverage, service delivery policies, and attitude toward both the professional and the client. Currently, there are four major methods of providing funds for service: (1) private insurers (including the nonprofit Blue Cross/Blue Shield and for-profit commercial insurers), (2) Medicare, (3) Medicaid, and (4) self pay.

1. Private Insurers

Managed Care. Managed medical care is strictly an outgrowth of the private sector. Since 1973 there has been a steady trend toward plans that require prepayment for anticipated services. Prepayment plans charge a fixed fee and the insuring organization then guarantees to provide a broad range of medical services with no additional fees. In an HMO or competitive medical plan (CMP), physicians share the risk of financing health care for an enrolled population. In return, physicians are offered a choice between billing and collecting a fee for service from the patient, or having the HMO pay the physician directly out of a prepaid per capita payment (capitation) for health care services. HMOs assume responsibility for providing a comprehensive range of health care services to voluntarily-enrolled populations at a fixed annual premium.

HMOs and CMPs contract with Medicare to provide services to Medicare beneficiaries. Under these contracts, a plan enrolls Medicare beneficiaries and is paid a predetermined monthly capitation payment by Medicare for each such individual. If the HMO or CMP provides services for less than the plan's capitation revenues, it keeps the residual as profits; if services to enrollees cost more than the capitation payments, the HMO or CMP loses money. Each participating HMO and CMP must provide, at a minimum, the same benefits that are otherwise available under Medicare, including both Part A and Part B benefits if the enrollee is eligible for both parts. These plans may, subject to certain limits, charge enrollees additional premiums, coinsurance, or copayment amounts. Persons enrolling in these plans agree to receive all covered services through the plans. Out-of-plan services are only covered on an emergency basis and are paid for by the HMO or CMP. Enrollees are liable for the cost of nonemergency out-of-plan services that have not been authorized by the HMO or CMP.

Nonprofit and Commercial Insurers. Blue Cross/Blue Shield is a nonprofit national association offering a variety of health insurance products. Since each state has its own Blue Cross/Blue Shield board, payment regulations vary from state to state. Therefore, it is necessary to determine the reimbursement categories allowed by the client's policy. Initially commercial insurers differed from the nonprofit Blue Cross/Blue Shield insurance in the manner in which the consumer received their benefits. Commercial insurers offered *indemnity benefits* (cash) while Blue Cross/Blue Shield offered *service benefits.* Although Blue Cross/Blue Shield was the first to offer health coverage, today many individuals are covered by private insurers other than Blue Cross/Blue Shield either through their place of work or individually. Benefits vary depending on the policy.

2. Medicare

Medicare is a nationwide insurance policy established by Congress in 1965. Medicare insurance is available to all citizens aged 65 and older, to certain disabled people under 65, and to people of any age with permanent kidney failure. Medicare is administered by the Health Care Finance Administration (HCFA). The Social Security Administration provides information about the program and handles enrollment. There are approximately 30 million aged and 3 million disabled individuals receiving Medicare benefits (Koitz, Reuter, & Merlis, 1989). There are two parts to the Medicare policy. In 1984,

97% of the population aged 65 and older was covered by one or both parts of Medicare (U.S. Department of Health and Human Services).

Part A. Part A, Hospital Insurance (HI), provides limited protection against the major costs arising from hospitalization. All Americans covered under the Social Security Administration or Railroad Retirement system must pay into the Medicare fund under the Federal Insurance Contributions Act (FICA) and Self-Employment Contributions Act (SECA). Enrollment in Part A is automatic for persons who are eligible. Part A is premium-free to qualified beneficiaries. Persons who do not have Social Security or Railroad Retirement benefits are not covered under Medicare Part A. However, married persons who do not have Social Security or Railroad Retirement benefits will be covered if their spouse is a qualified Medicare beneficiary (QMB). Persons who do not qualify for premium-free Part A benefits may buy the coverage if they meet certain requirements. As with most insurance policies, there are deductibles and coinsurance for Part A. Exhibit 11–1 shows the hospital insurance covered services for 1996.

Part B. Medicare Part B, supplemental medical insurance (SMI), is a separate and voluntary insurance program designed to provide limited protection against physician and certain other medical charges. The cost to the consumer for Part B is based on the statistics for the group using the program. Increases in medical bills reflect on the specific group involved in the program by raising the group members' monthly payments. When the program began in 1966, monthly premiums paid by enrollees were set in the law to finance half of the program's costs. The other half was to be paid for by the consumer. However, over the years the premium's growth did not keep pace with the rapidly rising costs of the program. As a result, the program currently receives only one-fourth of its financing from premiums. Unlike Part A, anyone aged 65 and older can elect to enroll in Part B. Exhibit 11–2 illustrates the medical insurance covered services for 1996.

Medigap. Medigap insurance is specifically designed to supplement Medicare's benefits. (See Exhibit 11–3 for gaps in coverage.) Although the policies are sold by commercial insurers, Medigap policies are regulated by federal and state law and must be clearly identified as Medicare supplement insurance. To make it easier for consumers to comparison shop for Medigap insurance, nearly all states limit the number of different Medigap policies that can be sold in that state to no more than ten standard plans, designated Plan A through Plan J, with Plan A being the most basic and Plan J the most comprehensive. The plans cover specific expenses either not covered or not fully covered by Medicare. Each state must allow the sale of Plan A and all Medigap insurers must make Plan A available if they are going to sell any Medigap plans in a state. Minnesota, Massachusetts, and Wisconsin had alternative Medigap standardization programs in effect before 1992, the year that federal legislation standardizing Medigap was enacted. These states, therefore were not required to change their Medigap plans to match the federal plans. For information on the Medigap plans in these states, contact that state's insurance department. Exhibit 11–4 is a chart of the ten standard Medicare supplement plans.

3. Medicaid

Medicaid is a joint federal-state health care program designed to provide health care for low-income individuals and families. Each state, using broad federal guidelines, establishes its own program of services and eligibility. In addition to the standard Medicaid program, there are two other programs available through state Medicaid offices, the QMB program and the Specified Low-Income Medicare Beneficiary (SLMB) program. These programs are designed specifically to help certain low-income Medicare beneficiaries meet their health care costs. The QMB program pays Medicare's premiums, deductibles, and coinsurance amounts for certain elderly and disabled persons who are entitled to

Exhibit 11–1 Medicare (Part A): Hospital Insurance Covered Services for 1996

Services	Benefit	Medicare Pays	You Pay
HOSPITALIZATION Semiprivate room and board, general nursing, and other hospital services and supplies. (Medicare payments based on benefit periods.)	First 60 days	All but $736	$736
	61st to 90th day	All but $184 a day	$184 a day
	91st to 150th day*	All but $368 a day	$368 a day
	Beyond 150 days	Nothing	All costs
SKILLED NURSING FACILITY CARE Semiprivate room and board, skilled nursing and rehabilitative services, and other services and supplies.** (Medicare coverage based on benefit periods.)	First 20 days	100% of approved amount	Nothing
	Additional 80 days	All but $92 a day	Up to $92 a day
	Beyond 100 days	Nothing	All costs
HOME HEALTH CARE Part-time or intermittent skilled care, home health aide services, durable medical equipment and supplies, and other services.	Unlimited as long as you meet Medicare requirements for home health care benefits.	100% of approved amount; 80% of approved amount for durable medical equipment.	Nothing for services; 20% of approved amount for durable medical equipment.
HOSPICE CARE Pain relief, symptom management, and support services for the terminally ill.	For as long as doctor certifies need.	All but limited costs for outpatient drugs and inpatient respite care.	Limited cost sharing for outpatient drugs and inpatient respite care.
BLOOD When furnished by a hospital or skilled nursing facility during a covered stay.	Unlimited during a benefit period if medically necessary.	All but first 3 pints per calendar year.	For first 3 pints.***

*   60 reserve days may be used only once.
**   Neither Medicare nor Medigap insurance will pay for most nursing home care.
***To the extent any of the three pints of blood are paid for or replaced under one part of Medicare during the calendar year, they do not have to be paid for or replaced under the other part.

Exhibit 11–2 Medicare (Part B): Medical Insurance Covered Services for 1996

Services	Benefit	Medicare Pays	You Pay
MEDICAL EXPENSES Physician's services, inpatient and outpatient medical and surgical services and supplies, physical and speech therapy, diagnostic tests, durable medical equipment, and other services.	Unlimited if medically necessary.	80% of approved amount (after $100 deductible). 50% of approved amount for most outpatient mental health services.	$100 deductible,* plus 20% of approved amount and limited charges above approved amount.** 50% for most mental health services.
CLINICAL LABORATORY SERVICES Blood tests, urinalysis, and more.	Unlimited if medically necessary.	Generally 100% of approved amount.	Nothing for services.
HOME HEALTH CARE Part-time or intermittent skilled care, home health aide services, durable medical equipment and supplies, and other services.	Unlimited as long as you meet Medicare requirements.	100% of approved amount; 80% of amount Medicare approves for durable medical equipment.	Nothing for services; 20% of amount Medicare approves for durable medical equipment.
OUTPATIENT HOSPITAL TREATMENT Services for the diagnosis or treatment of an illness or injury.	Unlimited if medically necessary.	Medicare payment to hospital based on hospital costs.	20% of billed amount (after $100 deductible).*
BLOOD	Unlimited if medically necessary.	80% of approved amount (after $100 deductible and starting with 4th pint).	First 3 pints plus 20% of approved amount for additional pints (after $100 deductible).***

* Once you have had $100 of expense for covered services, the Part B deductible does not apply to any other covered services you receive for the rest of the year.
** Federal law limits charges for physician services.
***To the extent any of the three pints of blood are paid for or replaced under one part of Medicare during the calendar year they do not have to be paid for or replaced under the other part.

Exhibit 11–3 Gaps In Doctor and Medical Supplier Coverage

Consumer must pay:

- $100 annual deductible.

- Generally, 20% coinsurance and permissible charges in excess of Medicare-approved amount.

- 50% of the Medicare-approved amounts for most outpatient mental health treatment.

- All charges in excess of Medicare's maximum yearly payment of $720 for independent physical or occupational therapists.

- All charges for most services that are not reasonable and necessary for the diagnosis or treatment of an illness or injury.

- All charges for most self-administerable prescription drugs and immunizations, except for pneumococcal, influenza, and hepatitis B vaccinations.

- All charges for routine physicals and other screening services, except for mammograms and Pap smears.

- All charges for routine eye examinations or eyeglasses, except prosthetic lenses after cataract surgery.

- All charges for acupuncture treatment.

- All charges for most dental care and dentures.

- All charges for hearing aids or routine hearing loss examinations.

- All charges for care outside the United States and its territories, except in certain instances in Canada and Mexico.

- All charges for routine foot care except when a medical condition affecting the lower limbs (such as diabetes) requires care by a medical professional.

- All charges for services of naturopaths, Christian Science practitioners, immediate relatives, or charges imposed by members of your household.

- Unless replaced, all charges for the first 3 pints of whole blood or units of packed cells used in each year in connection with covered services. To the extent the 3-pint blood deductible is met under Part A, it does not have to be met under Part B.

Medicare Part A, whose annual income is at or below the national poverty level, and whose savings are very limited. The QMB program functions like a Medigap policy and more because it pays the Part B premium and is not obligated to pay deductibles, coinsurance, and other related charges.

The SLMB program is for persons entitled to Medicare Part A but whose income is slightly higher than the QMB. In 1995, to qualify as a SLMB the recipient's income could not exceed 20% of the national poverty level. When a SLMB becomes a Medicaid recipient, federal law requires that each state pay for the Part B premiums. When a service is billed under Part B of Medicare, the SLMB is responsible for Medicare's deductibles, coinsurance, and other related charges.

4. Self Pay

Although there is little doubt that the availability of third-party payment helps to make any service more attractive, the presence or absence of insurance coverage should not determine whether or not a specific service is offered. Many clients who are not covered for services through insurance opt to pay for a needed service out of pocket.

Exhibit 11–4 Chart of the Ten Standard Medicare Supplement Plans

Medicare supplement insurance can be sold in only 10 standard plans. This chart shows the benefits included in each plan. Every company must make available Plan A. Some plans may not be available in your state.

Basic Benefits: Included in all plans.
Hospitalization: Part A coinsurance plus coverage for 365 additional days after Medicare benefits end.
Medical Expenses: Part B coinsurance (generally 20% of Medicare-approved expenses).
Blood: First 3 pints of blood each year.

A	B	C	D	E	F	G	H	I	J
Basic	Basic	Basic	Basic	Basic	Basic	Basic	Basic	Basic	Basic
		Skilled Nursing	Skilled Nursing	Skilled Nursing	Skilled Nursing	Skilled Nursing	Skilled Nursing	Skilled Nursing	Skilled Nursing
	Part A	Part A	Part A	Part A	Part A	Part A	Part A	Part A	Part A
		Part B			Part B				Part B
					Part B Excess	Part B Excess		Part B Excess	Part B Excess
		Foreign Travel	Foreign Travel	Foreign Travel	Foreign Travel	Foreign Travel	Foreign Travel	Foreign Travel	Foreign Travel
			At Home			At Home		At Home	At Home
							Basic Drug Benefit	Basic Drug Benefit	Extended Drug Benefit
				Preventive					Preventive

continues

Exhibit 11–4 continued

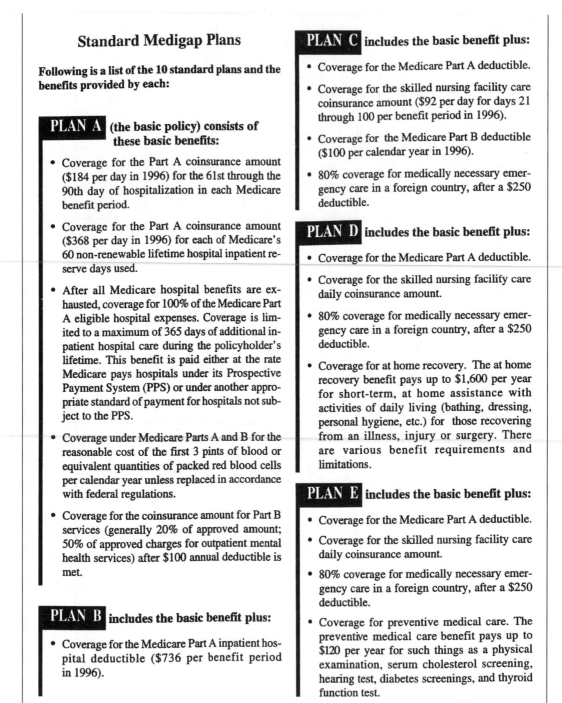

Standard Medigap Plans

Following is a list of the 10 standard plans and the benefits provided by each:

PLAN A (the basic policy) consists of these basic benefits:

- Coverage for the Part A coinsurance amount ($184 per day in 1996) for the 61st through the 90th day of hospitalization in each Medicare benefit period.

- Coverage for the Part A coinsurance amount ($368 per day in 1996) for each of Medicare's 60 non-renewable lifetime hospital inpatient reserve days used.

- After all Medicare hospital benefits are exhausted, coverage for 100% of the Medicare Part A eligible hospital expenses. Coverage is limited to a maximum of 365 days of additional inpatient hospital care during the policyholder's lifetime. This benefit is paid either at the rate Medicare pays hospitals under its Prospective Payment System (PPS) or under another appropriate standard of payment for hospitals not subject to the PPS.

- Coverage under Medicare Parts A and B for the reasonable cost of the first 3 pints of blood or equivalent quantities of packed red blood cells per calendar year unless replaced in accordance with federal regulations.

- Coverage for the coinsurance amount for Part B services (generally 20% of approved amount; 50% of approved charges for outpatient mental health services) after $100 annual deductible is met.

PLAN B includes the basic benefit plus:

- Coverage for the Medicare Part A inpatient hospital deductible ($736 per benefit period in 1996).

PLAN C includes the basic benefit plus:

- Coverage for the Medicare Part A deductible.

- Coverage for the skilled nursing facility care coinsurance amount ($92 per day for days 21 through 100 per benefit period in 1996).

- Coverage for the Medicare Part B deductible ($100 per calendar year in 1996).

- 80% coverage for medically necessary emergency care in a foreign country, after a $250 deductible.

PLAN D includes the basic benefit plus:

- Coverage for the Medicare Part A deductible.

- Coverage for the skilled nursing facility care daily coinsurance amount.

- 80% coverage for medically necessary emergency care in a foreign country, after a $250 deductible.

- Coverage for at home recovery. The at home recovery benefit pays up to $1,600 per year for short-term, at home assistance with activities of daily living (bathing, dressing, personal hygiene, etc.) for those recovering from an illness, injury or surgery. There are various benefit requirements and limitations.

PLAN E includes the basic benefit plus:

- Coverage for the Medicare Part A deductible.

- Coverage for the skilled nursing facility care daily coinsurance amount.

- 80% coverage for medically necessary emergency care in a foreign country, after a $250 deductible.

- Coverage for preventive medical care. The preventive medical care benefit pays up to $120 per year for such things as a physical examination, serum cholesterol screening, hearing test, diabetes screenings, and thyroid function test.

continues

Exhibit 11–4 continued

PLAN F includes the basic benefit plus:

- Coverage for the Medicare Part A deductible.

- Coverage for the skilled nursing facility care daily coinsurance amount.

- Coverage for the Medicare Part B deductible.

- 80% coverage for medically necessary emergency care in a foreign country, after a $250 deductible.

- Coverage for 100% of Medicare Part B excess charges.*

PLAN G includes the basic benefit plus:

- Coverage for the Medicare Part A deductible.

- Coverage for the skilled nursing facility care daily coinsurance amount.

- Coverage for 80% of Medicare Part B excess charges.*

- 80% coverage for medically necessary emergency care in a foreign country, after a $250 deductible.

- Coverage for at home recovery (see Plan D).

PLAN H includes the basic benefit plus:

- Coverage for the Medicare Part A deductible.

- Coverage for the skilled nursing facility care daily coinsurance amount.

- 80% coverage for medically necessary emergency care in a foreign country, after a $250 deductible.

- Coverage for 50% of the cost of prescription drugs up to a maximum annual benefit of $1,250 after the policyholder meets a $250 per year deductible (this is called the "basic" prescription drug benefit).

PLAN I includes the basic benefit plus:

- Coverage for the Medicare Part A deductible.

- Coverage for the skilled nursing facility care daily coinsurance amount.

- Coverage for 100% of Medicare Part B excess charges.*

- Basic prescription drug coverage (see Plan H for description).

- 80% coverage for medically necessary emergency care in a foreign country, after a $250 deductible.

- Coverage for at home recovery (see Plan D).

PLAN J includes the basic benefit plus:

- Coverage for the Medicare Part A deductible.

- Coverage for the skilled nursing facility care daily coinsurance amount.

- Coverage for the Medicare Part B deductible.

- Coverage for 100% of Medicare Part B excess charges.*

- 80% coverage for medically necessary emergency care in a foreign country, after a $250 deductible.

- Coverage for preventive medical care (see Plan E).

- Coverage for at home recovery (see Plan D).

- Coverage for 50% of the cost of prescription drugs up to a maximum annual benefit of $3,000 after the policyholder meets a $250 per year deductible (this is called the "extended" drug benefit).

* Plan pays a specified percentage of the difference between Medicare's approved amount for Part B services and the actual charges (up to the amount of charge limitations set by either Medicare or state law).

Tips for Reimbursement

The following general guidelines should be kept in mind when seeking reimbursement.

1. The facility or agency providing the service must be approved or certified by the insurance carrier to provide services.
2. The therapist must be qualified.
3. The patient or client must be eligible for benefits.
4. The therapist should know the policy details before initiating therapy.

MEDICARE REGULATIONS AFFECTING REIMBURSEMENT

Rehabilitation professionals are often asked to evaluate clients who are not candidates for ongoing treatment. Since 1981, Medicare regulations have recognized that persons entering nursing homes may be at risk for losing latent and/or dormant functional abilities that are not stimulated. In such cases, when the rehabilitation professional believes that the caregivers and the client need information gained during the initial evaluation to promote stimulation tasks, Medicare will reimburse the professional for his or her skilled services. The guideline states "... After the initial evaluation of the extent of the disorder or illness, if the restoration potential is judged insignificant or, after a reasonable period of trial, the patient's response to treatment is judged insignificant or at a plateau, an appropriate functional maintenance program may be established.... The initial evaluation of the patient's needs, the designing by the qualified speech pathologist of the maintenance program..., the instruction of the patient and supportive personnel (e.g., aides or nursing personnel, or family members...) in carrying out the program..." constitute a covered service (*Medicare Outpatient Physical Therapy Manual,* 1981, October).

The skilled nature of this service is established through the documentation of recommendations and instructions (see Unit 10). A specific reference pertaining to the type of documentation required for the establishment of a reimbursable maintenance program for persons with Alzheimer's disease can be found in the *Medicare Skilled Nursing Facility Manual* (1989, May), section 543.1 under *B. Maintenance.*

> I. **Alzheimer's Disease.** (Chronic brain syndrome, organic brain syndrome). Your objective documentation must indicate the patient's condition, alertness and mental awareness. Justify that services are needed for establishment of a maintenance program.

This section is repeated in the *Medicare Intermediary Manual,* Part 3, (1991, June) Claims Process.

A concern of some clinicians is the limitation of services allowed under Medicare for treatment of Alzheimer's due to the nature of the disease process. While there is clearly a limit on the amount of psychiatric treatment, this limit does not exist when the treatment is for medical or rehabilitative reasons other than those of a psychiatric nature. To this end, Medicare recognizes two separate ICD-9 codes for the disease, 290 (psychiatric) and 331 (medical) and states:

> 2476.2 **Diagnosis of Alzheimer's disease or a Related Disorder.** Where the primary diagnosis reported by the physician for a particular service is Alzheimer's disease (coded 331.0 in the *International Classification of Diseases (9th Rev.)* or Alzheimer's or other disorders coded 290.XX in the APA's *Diagnostic and Statistical Manual-Mental Disorders,* look to the nature of the service that has been rendered in determining whether it is subject to the benefit limitation. Typically, treatment provided a patient with a diagnosis of Alzheimer's disease or a related disorder will represent medical management of the patient's condition (rather than psychiatric treatment) and *will not* be subject to the benefit limitation. However, where a par-

ticular treatment rendered a patient with such a diagnosis is primarily psychotherapy, it *will* be subject to the limitation. (*Medicare Carriers Manual,* 1987, August)

To ensure coverage it is important that the clinician clearly indicate that treatment is not psychiatric in nature and use the appropriate ICD-9 code.

Another frequent question regarding reimbursement deals with the nature or type of service being provided. Therapists sometimes feel that if they have not done something hands on they will not be reimbursed. This is, of course, not the case as the Medicare Transmittal No. A-88-1 clearly states:

> 2. **Observation and Assessment of Patient Condition.** Observation and assessment are skilled services when the likelihood of change in a patient's condition requires skilled nursing or skilled rehabilitation personnel to identify and evaluate the patient's need for possible modification of treatment or initiation of additional medical procedures, until the patient's treatment regimen is essentially stabilized (Health Care Finance Administration, 1988, February).

The key words here are "skilled service." Although there are many services which may at first seem to be routine in nature, they may in fact be skilled and reimbursable because they require the skills of a therapist. An explanation of this key to reimbursement can be found in this same transmittal in section 3132.1 Skilled Nursing and Skilled Rehabilitation Services, which states in part "A skilled service means that a skilled person must be needed to perform the service *or* supervise its performance . . . ." The test is to ask oneself if the task (evaluating the patient, developing a program, etc.) requires the skills of the therapist. If the skills of a therapist are needed, then the task is a skilled service.

A complete copy of Transmittal No. A-88-1 can be found in Appendix 11–A. This transmittal is unusual in that it is in the form of instructions to the intermediaries. Those portions of the transmittal that appear in the boxes are instructions from HCFA to the intermediary with regard to coverage policy for skilled nursing facility reviews. Intermediaries are instructed to review *for coverage.* They are to look for evidence that services are covered based on the guidelines. Readers should note that this guideline clearly instructs the intermediary to "Address the services, not the diagnosis." With this thought in mind and the guidelines in hand, it is hoped that readers will no longer be timid about using "Alzheimer's" as a diagnosis worthy of treatment.

Changing Attitudes

Over the years, the necessity and efficacy of treating the Alzheimer's client have been attested to by the changes in Medicare treatment of outpatient visits. The 1984 Report of the Department of Health and Human Service's Task Force on Alzheimer's Disease recommended the removal of reimbursement limitations on certain outpatient physician services for Alzheimer's disease and related disorders. According to ADRDA, this recommendation was put into effect immediately by the Secretary of Health and Human Services.

Although this change in reimbursement is directed toward the need for psychiatric intervention and ongoing medical management provided by a psychiatrist, it recognizes the need for ongoing treatment by other disciplines as an auxiliary to medical care. It also opens the door to other needed disciplines and can be effective in assisting the client to achieve a better quality of life.

In this country, attitudes toward a particular disorder or disease are frequently reflected in the federal budget. For example, funding for dementia research increased steadily between 1976 and 1989. In 1976, when very little of the nation's attention was focused on Alzheimer's as a disease process, federal funds amounted to $4 million. By 1985, with Alzheimer's targeted as a disease to be reckoned with, the National Institutes of Health increased its Alzheimer's disease research budget to more than $50 million—a 50% increase over its 1984 budget. In 1989, the federal budget for dementia research was $120 million. In addition to basic research, in 1986, a House of Representatives committee approved legislation calling for a limited number of Medicare pilot projects. The projects were to support Alzheimer's clients' activities such as case management services, home and community-based services, outpatient drug therapy, respite care, and adult day care. In each case, Medicare covered the cost of providing services to participating clients. The majority of current research is funded by the National Institute on Aging (NIA), the Veterans Administration (VA), the National Institute of Neurological Disorders and Stroke (NINDS), and the National Institute of Mental Health (NIMH). Foundations and drug companies have provided additional funds.

Department of Health & Human Services—HCFA Memorandum BPO-043 Transmittal No. A-88-1 February 1988 Subject: Clarification of Part A Intermediary Transmittal No. 1365

SKILLED NURSING FACILITY CARE PURPOSE AND INTENT OF NEW GUIDELINES

The custodial care section of the manual has not been revised in 20 years. The SNF level of care section has not been revised for 12 years.

Beneficiaries, providers, and courts have grown increasingly displeased with what are perceived as inappropriate denials of SNF coverage.

We have revised and expanded the manual guidelines to present more clearly the requirements for coverage. The purpose is to make it easier to identify covered care and ensure that claims are approved when the requirements for coverage are met.

The SNF level of care guidelines and custodial care guidelines have been totally rewritten. The new description of custodial care eliminates outdated references to rehabilitation services. The new description of a covered level of SNF care presents a more detailed explanation of the three elements that must be met: skilled services, on a daily basis, that as a practical matter must be furnished in a SNF.

Approach to Level of Care Review

The guidelines are in a chapter titled COVERAGE OF SERVICES. Remember that you are reviewing for *coverage*. Look for evidence that services are covered, to approve the claim. If you can't find the evidence, then denial is appropriate. Do not approach a claim assuming it is noncovered and looking only for evidence to use in denying it.

When you use screens to focus your medical review efforts, they should be *coverage* screens. Cases that are screened out cannot be arbitrarily denied on level of care grounds just because they did not pass the screen. They must be developed and reviewed in more detail. In short, you can use medical review screens to approve claims without in-depth individual review, but not to deny them. Any rule of thumb that would declare the level of care requirements not met and deny a claim on the basis of elements such as the patient's condition, restoration potential, ability to walk, or degree of stability *without individual review of all pertinent facts to see if coverage could be justified* is unacceptable. A medical denial decision should be based on a detailed and thorough factual analysis of the patient's total condition and needs.

Custodial Care

This section has been revised dramatically. Most of the prior material has been eliminated. The more significant changes are

The discussion of skilled services has been deleted; cross reference is made to the SNF level of care sections in lieu of this.

The discussion of "primary purpose" has been eliminated. That material could be (and had been) misinterpreted to deny as "custodial" cases where daily skilled services were required. This section also had erroneously dismissed skilled rehabilitation services from consideration, and emphasized continuous nursing inappropriately.

The discussion of physicians' and ancillary services has been eliminated, as it no longer serves a useful purpose in this context.

A custodial care denial would be based on section 1862 (a)(9) of the law.

SNF Level of Care

Numerous examples are used to illustrate covered care. The emphasis is now placed on what *is* covered, rather than what should be denied.

The presentation closely follows the structure of the regulations, and reflects more accurately the coverage provisions of the statute and regulations.

A detailed discussion of skilled therapy, as a skilled rehabilitation service that can qualify a patient for SNF coverage, has been added.

Some presumptions that intermediaries may make have been added, which should help to simplify claims processing.

A level of care denial would be based on section 1862 (a)(1)(A) of the law.

Presentation of Training Materials

Using the new guidelines to decide whether an individual case is covered requires weighing the evidence and exercising judgment. The unique aspects of the individual patient often enter into the decision in several respects. In this training package, a star (★) has been placed at those parts of the guidelines where *individual case judgment* must be exercised.

For example, no star is shown at the entry under *Direct Skilled Nursing Services to Patients* which reads "Nasogastric tube, gastrostomy, and jejunostomy feedings." There is no room here for individual judgment about whether these services are skilled. These are *always* skilled nursing services. (Conceivably, one of these services might be given to a patient who does not require it. In that case, it could be denied as a *skilled service* that was not reasonable and necessary for the individual patient.)

In contrast, there is a star under the "practical matter" section to call attention to the necessity for deciding whether use of an available alternative source of care actually would be more economical in the individual case. This requirement cannot be evaluated without judging the facts for each individual patient.

For training purposes the new level of care guidelines are reproduced here (from the Intermediary Manual) with stars (as noted above) in the margin to indicate where individual case judgment is required, and with boxed *COMMENTS* inserted after important points to emphasize and illustrate them.

Following the guidelines are discussions of several issues that have been raised by readers.

COVERAGE OF SERVICES

3132. SKILLED NURSING FACILITY LEVEL OF CARE—GENERAL

Care in a SNF is covered if all of the following three factors are met:

- The patient requires skilled nursing services or skilled rehabilitation services, i.e., services that must be performed by or under the supervision of professional or technical personnel (see §§3132.1–3132.3);
- The patient requires these skilled services on a daily basis (see §3132.5); and
- As a practical matter, considering economy and efficiency, the daily skilled services can be provided only on an inpatient basis in an SNF. (See §3132.6.)

If any one of these three factors is not met, a stay in an SNF, even though it might include the delivery of some skilled services, is not covered. For example, payment for an SNF level of care could not be made if a patient needs an intermittent rather than daily skilled service.

In reviewing SNF services to determine whether the level of care requirements are met, first consider whether a patient needs skilled care. If a need for a skilled service does not exist, then the "daily" and "practical matter" requirements do not have to be addressed.

> FIRST, DECIDE IF ANY SKILLED NURSING OR SKILLED REHABILITATION SERVICES WERE NEEDED. IF YES, THEN DECIDE IF THOSE SKILLED SERVICES WERE DAILY. IF YES, THEN DECIDE IF THOSE DAILY SKILLED SERVICES AS A PRACTICAL MATTER COULD BE FURNISHED ONLY IN A SNF.

In addition, the services must be furnished pursuant to a physician's orders and be reasonable and necessary for the treatment of a patient's illness or injury, i.e., be consistent with the nature and severity of the individual's illness or injury, his particular medical needs, and accepted standards of medical practice. The services must also be reasonable in terms of duration and quantity.

EXAMPLE: Even though the irrigation of a catheter may be a skilled nursing service, daily irrigations may not be "reasonable and necessary" for the treatment of a patient's illness or injury.

> DECIDE IF THE DAILY SKILLED SERVICES ARE MEDICALLY APPROPRIATE FOR THE PATIENT.

3132.1 *Skilled Nursing and Skilled Rehabilitation Services*

A. *Skilled Services—Defined.*—Skilled nursing and/or skilled rehabilitation services are those services, furnished pursuant to physician orders, that:

- Require the skills of qualified technical or professional health personnel such as registered nurses, licensed practical (vocational) nurses, physical therapists, occupational therapists, and speech pathologists or audiologists; and
- Must be provided directly by or under the general supervision of these skilled nursing or skilled rehabilitation personnel to assure the safety of the patient and to achieve the medically desired result.

NOTE: "General supervision" requires initial direction and periodic inspection of the actual activity. However, the supervisor need not always be physically present or on the premises when the assistant is performing services.

Assume that skilled services provided by a participating SNF are furnished by or under the general supervision of the appropriate skilled nursing or skilled rehabilitation personnel.

> A SKILLED SERVICE MEANS THAT A SKILLED PERSON MUST BE NEEDED TO PERFORM THE SERVICE *OR* SUPERVISE ITS PERFORMANCE. SUPERVISION DOES NOT HAVE TO BE "OVER THE SHOULDER." DO NOT BASE COVERAGE DECISIONS ON WHETHER ACTUAL SUPERVISION WAS ADEQUATE. IF YOU HAVE EVIDENCE OF QUESTIONABLE SUPERVISION, REFER IT TO THE REGIONAL OFFICE FOR EXPLORATION BY THE STATE SURVEY AGENCY.

B. *Principles for Determining Whether a Service is Skilled*

> THESE GENERAL PRINCIPLES ARE IMPORTANT. READ THEM CAREFULLY. YOU CAN USE THEM TO DECIDE IF A SERVICE NOT MENTIONED IN THE GUIDELINES IS SKILLED. HOWEVER, IF A SERVICE IS IDENTIFIED IN THE GUIDELINES AS SKILLED, YOU *CANNOT* USE THESE PRINCIPLES TO DECIDE OTHERWISE. IN CONTRAST, AT TIMES YOU MUST USE THE PRINCIPLES TO DECIDE IF A SERVICE OR COMBINATION OF SERVICES THAT IS IDENTIFIED IN THE GUIDELINES AS USUALLY NONSKILLED ACTUALLY *IS* SKILLED IN A PARTICULAR CASE.

- If the inherent complexity of a service prescribed for a patient is such that it can be performed safely and/or effectively only by or under the general supervision of skilled nursing or skilled rehabilitation personnel, the service is a skilled service; e.g., the administration of intravenous feedings and intramuscular injections; the insertion of catheters; and ultrasound, shortwave, and microwave therapy treatments.

> SOME SERVICES, BY THEIR VERY NATURE, ALWAYS ARE SKILLED. EXAMPLES OF THESE ARE LISTED LATER, IN 3132.2 AND 3132.3A2.

- Consider the nature of the service and the skills required for safe and effective delivery of that service in deciding whether a service is a skilled service. While a patient's particular medical condition is a valid factor in deciding if skilled services are needed, a patient's diagnosis or prognosis should never be the sole factor in deciding that a service is not skilled.

EXAMPLE: Even where a patient's full or partial recovery is not possible, a skilled service still could be needed to prevent deterioration or to maintain current capabilities. A cancer patient, for instance, whose prognosis is terminal may require skilled services at various stages of his illness in connection with periodic "tapping" to relieve fluid accumulation and nursing assessment and intervention to alleviate pain or prevent deterioration. The fact that there is no potential for such a patient's recovery does not alter the character of the services and skills required for their performance.

When rehabilitation services are the primary services, the key issue is whether the skills of a therapist are needed. The deciding factor is not the patient's potential for recovery, but whether the services needed require the skills of a therapist or whether they can be carried out by nonskilled personnel. (See §3132.3.A.)

> OTHER SERVICES *MAY* BE SKILLED, DEPENDING ON WHAT IS ACTUALLY NEEDED. THE PATIENT'S CONDITION CAN INFLUENCE YOUR DECISION BECAUSE IT RELATES TO WHAT SKILLS ARE NEEDED. HOWEVER, AN ARBITRARY DENIAL SUCH AS "OLD STROKE: NONCOVERED" IS *NOT* SUPPORTABLE. ADDRESS THE SERVICES, NOT THE DIAGNOSIS.

- A service that is ordinarily considered nonskilled could be considered a skilled service in cases in which, because of special medical complications, skilled nursing or skilled rehabilitation personnel are required to perform or supervise it or to observe the patient. In these cases, the complications and special services involved must be documented by physicians' orders and nursing or therapy notes.

EXAMPLE: The existence of a plaster cast on an extremity generally does not indicate a need for skilled care. However, a patient with a preexisting acute skin problem, preexisting peripheral vascular disease, or a need for special traction of the injured extremity might need skilled nursing or skilled rehabilitation personnel to observe for complications or to adjust traction.

EXAMPLE: Whirlpool baths do not ordinarily require the skills of a qualified physical therapist. However, the skills, knowledge, and judgment of a qualified physical therapist might be required where the patient's condition is complicated by circulatory deficiency, areas of desensitization, or open wounds.

- In determining whether services rendered in an SNF constitute covered care, it is necessary to determine whether individual services are skilled, and whether, in light of the patient's total condition, skilled management of the services provided is needed even though many or all of the specific services were unskilled.

EXAMPLE: An 81-year-old woman who is aphasic and confused, suffers from hemiplegia, congestive heart failure, and atrial fibrillation, has suffered a cerebrovascular accident, is incontinent and has a Grade 1 decubitus ulcer, and is unable to communicate and make her needs known. Even though no specific service provided is skilled, the patient's condition requires daily skilled nursing involvement to manage a plan for the total care needed, to observe the patient's progress, and to evaluate the need for changes in the treatment plan.

> EVEN NONSKILLED SERVICES CAN, AT TIMES, REQUIRE SKILLS EITHER IN THEIR PERFORMANCE OR THEIR MANAGEMENT.

- The importance of a particular service to an individual patient, or the frequency with which it must be performed, does not, by itself, make it a skilled service.

EXAMPLE: A primary need of a nonambulatory patient may be frequent changes of position in order to avoid development of decubitus ulcers. However, since such changing of position does not ordinarily require skilled nursing or skilled rehabilitation personnel, it would not constitute a skilled service, even though such services are obviously necessary.

The possibility of adverse effects from the improper performance of an otherwise unskilled service does not make it a skilled service unless there is documentation to support the need for skilled nursing or skilled rehabilitation personnel. Although the act of turning a patient normally is not a skilled service, for some patients the skills of a nurse may be necessary to assure proper body alignment in order to avoid contractures and deformities. In all such cases, the reasons why skilled nursing or skilled rehabilitation personnel are essential must be documented in the patient's record.

> NECESSITY OF A SERVICE FOR A PATIENT'S WELL-BEING DOES NOT RELATE TO SKILLS. BASIC HUMAN NEEDS LIKE FOOD AND SHELTER ARE ESSENTIAL TO SUSTAIN LIFE, BUT DO NOT REQUIRE SKILLED HEALTH PERSONNEL TO FURNISH THEM.

C. *Specific Examples of Some Skilled Nursing or Skilled Rehabilitation Services*

1. **Management and Evaluation of a Patient Care Plan.**—The development, management, and evaluation of a patient care plan, based on the physician's orders, constitute skilled nursing services when, in terms of the patient's physical or mental condition, these services require the involvement of skilled nursing personnel to meet the patient's medical needs, promote recovery, and ensure medical safety. However, the planning and management of a treatment plan that does not involve the furnishing of skilled services may not require skilled nursing personnel. Skilled management would be required where the sum total of unskilled services which are a necessary part of the medical regimen, when considered in light of the patient's overall condition, makes the involvement of skilled nursing personnel necessary to promote the patient's recovery and medical safety.

EXAMPLE 1: An aged patient with a history of diabetes mellitus and angina pectoris is recovering from an open reduction of the neck of the femur. He requires, among other services, careful skin care, appropriate oral medications, a diabetic diet, a therapeutic exercise program to preserve muscle tone and body condition, and observation to notice signs of deterioration in his condition or complications resulting from his restricted (but increasing) mobility. Although any of the required services could be performed by a properly instructed person, that person would not have the capability to understand the relationship among the services and their effect on each other. Since the nature of the patient's condition, his age and his immobility create a high potential for serious complications, such an understanding is essential to assure the patient's recovery and safety. The management of this plan of care requires skilled nursing personnel until the individual services involved are supportive in nature and do not require skilled nursing personnel.

EXAMPLE 2: An aged patient is recovering from pneumonia, is lethargic, is disoriented, has residual chest congestion, is confined to bed as a result of his debilitated condition, and requires restraints at times. To decrease the chest congestion, the physician has prescribed frequent changes in position, coughing, and deep breathing. While the residual chest congestion alone would not represent a high risk factor, the patient's immobility and confusion represent complicating factors which, when coupled with the chest congestion, could create high probability of a relapse. In this situation, skilled overseeing of the nonskilled services would be reasonable and necessary, pending the elimination of the chest congestion, to assure the patient's medical safety.

> SKILLED SERVICES CAN BE NEEDED TO MANAGE CARE, DEPENDING ON THE PATIENT'S CONDITION. THIS DOES NOT SAY THAT *ALL* PATIENTS REQUIRE SKILLED MANAGEMENT, OR THAT IF IT IS NEEDED AT FIRST THE NEED CONTINUES INDEFINITELY. YOU MUST USE JUDGMENT TO DECIDE WHICH PATIENTS DO NEED SKILLED MANAGEMENT AND FOR HOW LONG.

Skilled planning and management activities are not always specifically identified in the patient's clinical record. Therefore, if the patient's overall condition supports a finding that recovery and safety can be assured only if the total care, skilled or not, is planned and managed by skilled nursing personnel, assume that skilled management is being provided even though it is not readily discernible from the record. Make this assumption only if the record as a whole clearly establishes that there was a likely potential for serious complications without skilled management.

> ACTUAL MANAGEMENT DOES NOT HAVE TO BE EXPLICITLY DOCUMENTED IF THE NEED FOR IT IS CLEAR IN THE RECORD. THE RECORD MUST REFLECT THE PATIENT'S CONDITION, TREATMENT REGIMEN, AND MEDICAL NEEDS, AND MUST CONTAIN EVIDENCE OF THE POTENTIAL FOR SERIOUS COMPLICATIONS, SO THAT YOU CAN EVALUATE WHETHER SKILLED MANAGEMENT WAS NEEDED.

2. *Observation and Assessment of Patient's Condition.*—Observation and assessment are skilled services when the likelihood of change in a patient's condition requires skilled nursing or skilled rehabilitation personnel to identify and evaluate the patient's need for possible modification of treatment or initiation of additional medical procedures, until the patient's treatment regimen is essentially stabilized.

EXAMPLE 1: A patient with arteriosclerotic heart disease with congestive heart failure requires close observation by skilled nursing personnel for signs of decompensation, abnormal fluid balance, or adverse effects resulting from prescribed medication. Skilled observation is needed to determine whether the digitalis dosage should be reviewed or whether other therapeutic measures should be considered, until the patient's treatment regimen is essentially stabilized.

EXAMPLE 2: A patient has undergone peripheral vascular disease treatment including revascularization procedures (bypass) with open or necrotic areas of skin on the involved extremity. Skilled observation and monitoring of the vascular supply of the legs is required.

EXAMPLE 3: A patient has undergone hip surgery and has been transferred to an SNF. Skilled observation and monitoring of the patient for possible adverse reaction to the operative procedure, development of phlebitis, skin breakdown, or need for the administration of subcutaneous Heparin, is both reasonable and necessary.

EXAMPLE 4: A patient has been hospitalized following a heart attack and, following treatment but before mobilization, is transferred to the SNF. Because it is unknown whether exertion will exacerbate the heart disease, skilled observation is reasonable and necessary as mobilization is initiated, until the patient's treatment regimen is essentially stabilized.

EXAMPLE 5: A frail 85-year-old man was hospitalized for pneumonia. The infection was resolved, but the patient, who had previously maintained adequate nutrition, will not eat or eats poorly. The patient is transferred to an SNF for monitoring of fluid and nutrient intake, assessment of the need for tube feeding and forced feeding if required. Observation and monitoring by skilled nursing personnel of the patient's oral intake is required to prevent dehydration.

> SKILLED OBSERVATION CAN BE NEEDED UNTIL THE *TREATMENT REGIMEN* IS ESSENTIALLY STABILIZED. YOU SHOULD LOOK FOR INDICATIONS IN THE RECORD THAT THE PHYSICIAN THINKS THE PATIENT'S CONDITION IS LIKELY TO CHANGE (A FURTHER ACUTE EPISODE OR COMPLICATION IS PROBABLE) AND OBSERVATION/ASSESSMENT IS NEEDED TO SEE IF THE TREATMENT SHOULD BE CHANGED. DO NOT CONFUSE STABILIZATION OF THE TREATMENT REGIMEN WITH STABILIZATION OF VITAL SIGNS. YOU MUST USE JUDGMENT TO DECIDE WHICH PATIENTS NEED OBSERVATION/ASSESSMENT, HOW FREQUENTLY THEY NEED IT (E.G., DAILY?), AND FOR HOW LONG.

If a patient was admitted for skilled observation but did not develop a further acute episode or complication, the skilled observation services still are covered so long as there was a reasonable probability for such a complication or further acute episode. "Reasonable probability" means that a potential complication or further acute episode was a likely possibility.

> DENIAL IS NOT APPROPRIATE JUST BECAUSE THE POTENTIAL DID NOT ACTUALLY OCCUR, SO LONG AS IT WAS *LIKELY* TO OCCUR.

Skilled observation and assessment may also be required for patients whose primary condition and needs are psychiatric in nature or for patients who, in addition to their physical problems, have a secondary psychiatric diagnosis. These patients may exhibit acute psychological symptoms such as depression, anxiety or agitation, which require skilled observation and assessment such as observing for indications of suicidal or hostile behavior. However, these conditions often require considerably more specialized, sophisticated nursing techniques and physician attention than is available in most participating SNFs. (SNFs that are primarily engaged in treating psychiatric disorders are precluded by law from participating in Medicare.) Therefore, these cases must be carefully documented.

> THE PURPOSE OF NURSING OBSERVATION AND ASSESSMENT IN THESE PSYCHIATRIC CASES IS TO IDENTIFY THE POTENTIAL FOR HARMFUL BEHAVIOR.

3. *Teaching and Training Activities.*—Teaching and training activities which require skilled nursing or skilled rehabilitation personnel to teach a patient how to manage his treatment regimen would constitute skilled services. Some examples are:

   - Teaching self-administration of injectable medications or a complex range of medications;

   - Teaching a newly diagnosed diabetic to administer insulin injections, to prepare and follow a diabetic diet, and to observe foot-care precautions;

   - Teaching self-administration of medical gases to a patient;

   - Gait training and teaching of prosthesis care for a patient who has had a recent leg amputation;

   - Teaching patients how to care for a recent colostomy or ileostomy;

   - Teaching patients how to perform self-catherization and self-administration of gastrostomy feedings;

   - Teaching patients how to care for and maintain central venous lines, such as Hickman catheters;

   - Teaching patients the use and care of braces, splints and orthotics, and any associated skin care; and

   - Teaching patients the proper care of any specialized dressings or skin treatments.

> SKILLED TEACHING OF SELF-CARE IS OFTEN A PART OF THE PERFORMANCE OF OTHER SKILLED SERVICES. NOTE THAT IN THIS LIST THE *TEACHING*, ITSELF, IS THE SKILLED SERVICE. THE ACTIVITY BEING TAUGHT MAY OR MAY NOT BE CONSIDERED SKILLED. REFER TO OTHER PARTS OF THE GUIDELINES TO SEE IF THE ACTIVITY IS SKILLED WHEN THE PATIENT DOES NOT PERFORM IT (FOR EXAMPLE, INSULIN INJECTIONS ARE DISCUSSED IN 3132.2, BELOW).

D. *Questionable Situations.*—There must be specific evidence that daily skilled nursing or skilled rehabilitation services are required and received if:

- The primary service needed is oral medication; or

- The patient is capable of independent ambulation, dressing, feeding, and hygiene.

> THIS LIST HAS BEEN SHORTENED CONSIDERABLY FROM THE PRIOR INSTRUCTION.

3132.2   Direct Skilled Nursing Services to Patients.—Some examples of direct skilled nursing services are:

- Intravenous, intramuscular or subcutaneous injections and hypodermoclysis or intravenous feeding (although giving an insulin injection is considered a skilled service, it is customary to teach patients to self-administer such an injection; if self-injection cannot be learned, however, insulin injection is a skilled service);

- Nasogastric tube, gastrostomy, and jejunostomy feedings;

- Naso-pharyngeal and tracheotomy aspiration;

- Insertion, sterile irrigation, and replacement of catheters; care of a suprapubic catheter and, in selected patients, urethral catheter (the mere presence of a urethral catheter, particularly one placed for convenience or the control of incontinence, does not justify a need for skilled nursing care. On the other hand, the insertion and maintenance of a urethral catheter as an adjunct to the active treatment of disease of the urinary tract may justify a need for skilled nursing care. In such instances, the need for a urethral catheter must be justified and documented in the patient's medical record; i.e., it must be established that it is reasonable and necessary for the treatment of the patient's condition.);

> THESE CATHETER CARE SERVICES *ARE* SKILLED. BUT THEY ALSO MUST BE REASONABLE AND NECESSARY FOR THE PATIENT. (SEE 3132.) THERE ARE TWO ASPECTS OF URETHRAL CATHETER CARE THAT MAY BE PROBLEMATIC. YOU MUST DETERMINE IF SUCH A CATHETER IS NEEDED, AND, IF IT IS, YOU MUST DETERMINE HOW FREQUENTLY STERILE IRRIGATION IS *NEEDED*. ANY SKILLED SERVICES THAT EXCEED THE PATIENT'S NEEDS WOULD BE DENIED AS NOT REASONABLE AND NECESSARY.

- Application of dressings involving prescription medications and aseptic techniques (see §3132.4 for exception);

- Treatment of decubitus ulcers, of a severity rated at Grade 3 or worse, or a widespread skin disorder (see §3132.4 for exception);

A GRADE 3 DECUBITUS ULCER IS DEFINED IN *THE MERCK MANUAL* AS "THE SKIN BECOMES NECROTIC, WITH EXPOSURE OF FAT." OTHER SOURCES USE SIMILAR DEFINITIONS FOR STAGE 3 OR GRADE III. THIS IS IN CONTRAST TO GRADE 2, WHICH "SHOWS REDNESS, EDEMA, AND INDURATION, AT TIMES WITH EPIDERMAL BLISTERING OR DESQUAMATION."

- Heat treatments which have been specifically ordered by a physician as part of active treatment and which require observation by skilled nursing personnel to adequately evaluate the patient's progress (see §3132.4 for exception);

- Rehabilitation nursing procedures, including the related teaching and adaptive aspects of nursing, that are part of active treatment and require the presence of skilled nursing personnel; e.g., the institution and supervision of bowel and bladder training programs;

- Initial phases of a regimen involving administration of medical gases such as bronchodilator therapy; and

- Care of a colostomy during the early postoperative period in the presence of associated complications. The need for skilled nursing care during this period must be justified and documented in the patient's medical record.

ALL OF THESE SERVICES *ARE* SKILLED, BY DEFINITION. IT IS NOT POSSIBLE TO DENY ANY OF THESE SERVICES AS UNSKILLED. HOWEVER, A SKILLED SERVICE THAT IS NOT NEEDED SHOULD BE DENIED AS NOT REASONABLE AND NECESSARY.

3132.3 Direct Skilled Rehabilitation Services to Patients

A. Skilled Physical Therapy

   1. General.—Skilled physical therapy services must meet all of the following conditions:

- The services must be directly and specifically related to an active written treatment plan designed by the physician after any needed consultation with a qualified physical therapist;

- The services must be of a level of complexity and sophistication, or the condition of the patient must be of a nature that requires the judgment, knowledge, and skills of a qualified physical therapist;

- The services must be provided with the expectation, based on the assessment made by the physician of the patient's restoration potential, that the condition of the patient will improve materially in a resonable and generally predictable period of time, or the services must be necessary for the establishment of a safe and effective maintenance program;

> SEE THE DISCUSSION OF REHABILITATION POTENTIAL FOLLOWING THESE GUIDELINES.

- The services must be considered under accepted standards of medical practice to be specific and effective treatment for the patient's condition; and

- The services must be reasonable and necessary for the treatment of the patient's condition; this includes the requirement that the amount, frequency, and duration of the services must be reasonable.

> THIS DEFINITION OF SKILLED PHYSICAL THERAPY, INCLUDING THE REST OF THE SECTION THAT FOLLOWS, PARALLELS THE STANDARD DEFINITION FOR OTHER PROGRAM PURPOSES, BUT HAS BEEN EDITED AND TAILORED FOR THE SNF LEVEL OF CARE CONTEXT.

EXAMPLE 1: An 80-year-old, previously ambulatory, post-surgical patient has been bedbound for one week and, as a result, has developed muscle atrophy, orthostatic hypotension, joint stiffness, and lower extremity edema. To the extent that the patient requires a brief period of daily skilled physical therapy services to restore lost functions, those services are reasonable and necessary.

EXAMPLE 2: A patient with congestive heart failure also has diabetes and previously had both legs amputated above the knees. Consequently, the patient does not have a reasonable potential to achieve ambulation, but still requires daily skilled physical therapy to learn bed mobility and transferring skills, as well as functional activities at the wheelchair level. If the patient has a reasonable potential for achieving those functions in a reasonable period of time in view of the patient's total condition, the physical therapy services are reasonable and necessary.

> THESE 2 EXAMPLES, WHILE NOT INCLUDED IN PREVIOUS HCFA GUIDELINES FOR PHYSICAL THERAPY COVERAGE IN OTHER SETTINGS, ARE FULLY CONSISTENT WITH THOSE INSTRUCTIONS. THE EXAMPLES ARE QUITE NARROW AND LIMITED; THEY DO NOT REFLECT AN EXPANSION IN THE SCOPE OF COVERAGE. THE FIRST EXAMPLE DOES NOT REPRESENT GENERALIZED "DECONDITIONING," BUT SPECIFIC NEUROLOGICAL, MUSCULAR, AND SKELETAL PROBLEMS. THE SECOND EXAMPLE SHOWS A RECENT AMPUTEE WHO NEEDS TO LEARN AND HAS THE POTENTIAL TO LEARN BED MOBILITY, TRANSFER SKILLS, AND WHEELCHAIR ACTIVITIES. WHILE BOTH EXAMPLES SHOW THAT SOME SKILLED PHYSICAL THERAPY CAN BE NEEDED BY SUCH PATIENTS, THE SKILLED SERVICES MUST BE *NEEDED* AND FURNISHED DAILY FOR SNF COVERAGE. YOU MUST USE YOUR JUDGMENT TO DETERMINE IF THE AMOUNT, FREQUENCY, AND DURATION ARE REASONABLE. ANY SKILLED SERVICES THAT EXCEED THE PATIENT'S NEEDS WOULD BE DENIED AS NOT REASONABLE AND NECESSARY.

If the expected results are insignificant in relation to the extent and duration of physical therapy services that would be required to achieve those results, the physical therapy would not be reasonable and necessary, and thus would not be covered skilled physical therapy services.

> USE CAREFUL JUDGMENT TO WEIGH EFFORTS NEEDED AGAINST THE ANTICI-
> PATED RESULTS. HOWEVER, DO NOT BASE THE DECISION ON *ACTUAL*
> RESULTS. THE TEST IS WHETHER IT WAS REASONABLE TO *EXPECT* SIGNIFI-
> CANT RESULTS.

Many SNF inpatients do not require skilled physical services but do require services which are routine in nature. Those services can be performed by supportive personnel; e.g., aides or nursing personnel, without the supervision of a physical therapist. Such services, as well as services involving activities for the general good and welfare of patients (e.g., general exercises to promote overall fitness and flexibility and activities to provide diversion or general motivation) do not constitute skilled physical therapy.

> THESE ROUTINE SERVICES CAN BE COVERED AS *PART OF* INPATIENT SNF CARE,
> BUT THEY DO *NOT* QUALIFY A PATIENT FOR A SNF LEVEL OF CARE BECAUSE
> THEY ARE NOT SKILLED SERVICES.

2. *Application of Guidelines.*—Some of the more common physical therapy modalities and procedures are:
   a. *Assessment.*—The skills of a physical therapist are required for the ongoing assessment of a patient's rehabilitation needs and potential. Skilled rehabilitation services concurrent with the management of a patient's care plan include tests and measurements of range of motion, strength, balance, coordination, endurance, and functional ability.
   b. *Therapeutic Exercises.*—Therapeutic exercises which must be performed by or under the supervision of the qualified physical therapist, due either to the type of exercise employed or to the condition of the patient, constitute skilled physical therapy.

> CONTRAST THIS AND THE FOLLOWING ACTIVITIES WITH THE DISCUSSION AT
> THE END OF 3132.4 ABOUT REPETITIOUS EXERCISES. DECIDING WHETHER A
> PARTICULAR ACTIVITY FOR A PARTICULAR PATIENT IS SKILLED WILL REQUIRE
> CAREFUL JUDGMENT.

   c. *Gait Training.*—Gait evaluation and training furnished a patient whose ability to walk has been impaired by neurological, muscular, or skeletal abnormality require the skills of a qualified physical therapist and constitute skilled physical therapy if they reasonably can be expected to improve significantly the patient's ability to walk.

Repetitious exercises to improve gait, or to maintain strength and endurance, and assistive walking are appropriately provided by supportive personnel, e.g., aides or nursing personnel, and do not require the skills of a physical therapist. Thus, such services are not skilled physical therapy.

> NOTE THAT A PATIENT'S ABILITY, FOR EXAMPLE, TO WALK WITH THE ASSISTANCE OF A WALKER OR CRUTCHES FOR UP TO 50 FEET SHOULD NEVER BE THE SOLE BASIS FOR DECIDING WHETHER THE PATIENT NEEDS SKILLED PHYSICAL THERAPY. SUCH A DECISION MUST BE BASED ON AN EVALUATION OF *ALL* RELEVANT FACTORS, AS DESCRIBED ABOVE IN 3132.3.A.1.

    d. *Range of Motion.*—Only the qualified physical therapist may perform range of motion tests and, therefore, such *tests* are skilled physical therapy. Range of motion *exercises* constitute skilled physical therapy only if they are part of active treatment for a specific disease state which has resulted in a loss or restriction of mobility (as evidenced by physical therapy notes showing the degree of motion lost and the degree to be restored).

Range of motion exercises which are not related to the restoration of a specific loss of function often may be provided safely by supportive personnel, such as aides or nursing personnel, and may not require the skills of a physical therapist. Passive exercises to maintain range of motion in paralyzed extremities that can be carried out by aides or nursing personnel would not be considered skilled care.

    e. *Maintenance Therapy.*—The repetitive services required to maintain function sometimes involve the use of complex and sophisticated therapy procedures and, consequently, the judgment and skill of a physical therapist might be required for the safe and effective rendition of such services. (See §3132.1.B.) The specialized knowledge and judgment of a qualified physical therapist may be required to establish a maintenance program intended to prevent or minimize deterioration caused by a medical condition, if the program is to be safely carried out and the treatment aims of the physician achieved. Establishing such a program is a skilled service.

EXAMPLE: A Parkinson's patient who has not been under a restorative physical therapy program may require the services of a physical therapist to determine what type of exercises are required for the maintenance of his present level of function. The initial evaluation of the patient's needs, the designing of a maintenance program which is appropriate to the capacity and tolerance of the patient and the treatment objectives of the physician, the instruction of the patient or supportive personnel (e.g., aides or nursing personnel) in the carrying out of the program, and such infrequent reevaluations as may be required, would constitute skilled physical therapy.

While a patient is under a restorative physical therapy program, the physical therapist should regularly reevaluate his condition and adjust any exercise program the patient is expected to carry out himself or with the aid of supportive personnel to maintain the function being restored. Consequently, by the time it is determined that no further restoration is possible, i.e., by the end of the last restorative session, the physical therapist will have already designed the maintenance program required and instructed the patient or supportive personnel in the carrying out of the program.

> MAINTENANCE IS A HIGHLY CONTROVERSIAL TOPIC. DESIGNING A MAINTE-
> NANCE PROGRAM REQUIRES SKILLS, BUT CARRYING IT OUT IS SKILLED
> ONLY IF A SPECIAL MEDICAL COMPLICATION EXISTS AND IS DOCUMENTED
> THAT MAKES SKILLED PERFORMANCE NECESSARY. AS NOTED IN THE NEXT
> SECTION, PERFORMANCE OR GENERAL SUPERVISION OF REPETITIVE EXER-
> CISES IS NONSKILLED.

f. *Ultrasound, Shortwave, and Microwave Diathermy Treatments.*—These modalities must always be performed by or under the supervision of a qualified physical therapist and are skilled physical therapy.

g. *Hot Packs, Infra-Red Treatments, Paraffin Baths and Whirlpool Baths.*—Heat treatments and baths of this type ordinarily do not require the skills of a qualified physical therapist. However, the skills, knowledge, and judgment of a qualified physical therapist might be required in the giving of such treatments or baths in a particular case, e.g., where the patient's condition is complicated by circulatory deficiency, areas of desensitization, open wounds, fractures or other complications.

> JUDGMENT IS NEEDED TO DECIDE WHETHER A PATIENT'S COMPLICATIONS
> REQUIRE THE SKILLS OF A PHYSICAL THERAPIST IN GIVING HEAT TREAT-
> MENTS AND BATHS. SEE THE DISCUSSION OF HEAT TREATMENTS IN 3132.2
> AND 3132.4.

B. *Speech Pathology.*—See §3101.10A.

C. *Occupational Therapy.*—See §3101.9.

3132.4 *Nonskilled Supportive or Personal Care Services.*—The following services are not skilled services unless rendered under circumstances detailed in §3132.1.B:

- Administration of routine oral medications, eye drops, and ointments (the fact that a patient cannot be relied upon to take such medications himself or that State law requires all medications to be dispensed by a nurse to institutional patients would not change this service to a skilled service);

- General maintenence care of colostomy and ileostomy;

- Routine services to maintain satisfactory functioning of indwelling bladder catheters (this would include emptying containers and cleaning them, and clamping tubing);

- Changes of dressings for noninfected postoperative or chronic conditions;

- Prophylactic and palliative skin care, including bathing and application of creams, or treatment of minor skin problems;

- Routine care of the incontinent patient, including use of diapers and protective sheets;

- General maintenance care in connection with a plaster cast (skilled supervision or observation may be required where the patient has a preexisting skin or circulatory condition or needs to have traction adjusted);

- Routine care in connection with braces and similar devices;

- Use of heat as a palliative and comfort measure, such as whirlpool or steam pack;

- Routine administration of medical gases after a regimen of therapy has been established (i.e., administration of medical gases after the patient has been taught how to institute therapy);

- Assistance in dressing, eating, and going to the toilet;

- Periodic turning and positioning in bed; and

- General supervision of exercises which have been taught to the patient and the performance of repetitious exercises that do not require skilled rehabilitation personnel for their performance. (This includes the actual carrying out of maintenance programs where the performance of repetitive exercises that may be required to maintain function do not necessitate a need for the involvement and services of skilled rehabilitation personnel. It also includes the carrying out of repetitive exercises to improve gait, maintain strength or endurance; passive exercises to maintain range of motion in paralyzed extremities which are not related to a specific loss of function; and assistive walking.) (See §3101.8D.)

> EACH OF THESE SUPPORTIVE SERVICES IS *NORMALLY* NOT SKILLED. THEY STILL CAN BE COVERED AS *PART OF* INPATIENT SNF CARE, BUT THEY DO NOT QUALIFY A PATIENT FOR A SNF LEVEL OF CARE UNLESS A DOCUMENTED SPECIAL MEDICAL COMPLICATION MAKES SKILLED PERFORMANCE NECESSARY.

3132.5   *Daily Skilled Services—Defined.*—Skilled nursing services or skilled rehabilitation services (or a combination of these services) must be needed and provided on a "daily basis," i.e., on essentially a 7-day-a-week basis. However, if skilled rehabilitation services are not available on a 7-day-a-week basis, a patient whose inpatient stay is based solely on the need for skilled rehabilitation services would meet the "daily basis" requirement when he needs and receives those services on at least 5 days a week. Accordingly, if a facility provides physical therapy on only 5 days a week and a patient in the facility requires and receives physical therapy on each of those days, the requirement that skilled rehabilitation services be provided on a daily basis is met. (If the services are available less than 5 days a week, though, the "daily" requirement would not be met.)

 This requirement should not be applied so strictly that it would not be met merely because there is an isolated break of a day or two during which no skilled rehabilitation services are furnished and discharge from the facility would not be practical.

EXAMPLE: A patient who normally requires skilled rehabilitation services on a daily basis may exhibit extreme fatigue that results in suspending therapy sessions for a day or two. Coverage may continue for these days since discharge in such a case would not be practical.

> ONCE YOU HAVE CONCLUDED THAT SKILLED SERVICES WERE NEEDED, THE NEXT STEP IS TO DECIDE WHETHER THOSE SERVICES WERE NEEDED AND FURNISHED DAILY. THIS SECTION IS VIRTUALLY UNCHANGED FROM THE PRIOR INSTRUCTION. ONE CLARIFICATION IS THAT A COMBINATION OF SKILLED SERVICES (SUCH AS PT ON MONDAY, WEDNESDAY, AND FRIDAY AND NURSING ON TUESDAY, THURSDAY, SATURDAY, AND SUNDAY) MEETS THE "DAILY" DEFINITION.

3132.6   *Services Provided on an Inpatient Basis as a "Practical Matter".*—In determining whether the daily skilled care needed by an individual can, as a "practical matter," only be provided in an SNF on an inpatient basis, consider the individual's physical condition and the availability and feasibility of using more economical alternative facilities or services.

> ONLY AFTER YOU HAVE DECIDED THAT DAILY SKILLED SERVICES WERE NEEDED AND FURNISHED DOES THE ISSUE OF "PRACTICAL MATTER" ARISE. NO MATTER WHAT SERVICES A PATIENT NEEDS NOR HOW DESPERATELY THEY ARE NEEDED, COVERAGE IN A SNF IS POSSIBLE ONLY IF THE SERVICES ARE BOTH *SKILLED* AND *DAILY*. YOU MUST FIND THAT SERVICES *ARE* SKILLED, AND ARE DAILY, TO JUSTIFY COVERAGE. THE "PRACTICAL MATTER" REQUIRE-MENT, HOWEVER, IS APPROACHED THE OPPOSITE WAY. ABSENT EVIDENCE TO THE CONTRARY, YOU WOULD ASSUME THAT THE REQUIREMENT IS MET. MOST CASES PROBABLY WILL NOT REQUIRE INDEPTH EXPLORATION BECAUSE IT WILL BE OBVIOUS THAT ALTERNATIVES TO SNF CARE ARE NOT PRACTICAL. IF YOU HAVE REASON TO THINK THAT THERE IS AN EQUALLY EFFECTIVE ALTER-NATIVE WHICH MIGHT BE PRACTICAL, EXAMINE AND DOCUMENT WHETHER, IN VIEW OF THE PATIENT'S CONDITION, THE ALTERNATIVE IS:
> *AVAILABLE,*
> *MORE ECONOMICAL,* AND
> *FEASIBLE.*

As a "practical matter," daily skilled services can be provided only in an SNF if they are not available on an outpatient basis in the area in which the individual resides or transportation to the closest facility would be:

- An excessive physical hardship;

- Less economical; or

- Less efficient or effective than an inpatient institutional setting.

The availability at home of capable and willing family or the feasibility of obtaining other assistance for the patient should be considered. Even though needed daily skilled services might be available on an outpatient or home care basis, as a practical matter, the care can be furnished only in the SNF if home care would be ineffective because the patient would have insufficient assistance at home to reside there safely.

EXAMPLE: A patient undergoing restorative physical therapy can walk only with supervision but has a reasonable potential to learn to walk independently with further training. Further daily skilled therapy is available on an outpatient or home care basis, but the patient would be at risk of further injury from falling, of dehydration or of malnutrition because insufficient supervision or assistance could be arranged for the patient in his home. In these circumstances, the physical therapy services as a practical matter can be provided effectively only in the inpatient setting.

> NOTE THAT THE ONLY ALTERNATIVES CITED ARE OUTPATIENT OR HOME CARE. INPATIENT (INSTITUTIONAL) CARE IS *NOT* A PRACTICAL ALTERNATIVE. IF A PATIENT NEEDS DAILY SKILLED SERVICES THAT MUST BE FURNISHED ON AN INPATIENT BASIS IT IS NEVER FEASIBLE, AS A PRACTICAL MATTER, TO PROVIDE THEM IN AN INSTITUTION OTHER THAN A MEDICARE PARTICIPATING SNF. IF THE SERVICES COULD BE PROVIDED OUTSIDE AN INSTITUTION, THE EFFECTIVENESS OF PROVIDING THEM IN THAT SETTING MAY DEPEND ON WHETHER ADEQUATE ASSISTANCE IS AVAILABLE.

A. *The Availability of Alternative Facilities or Services.*—Alternative facilities or services may be available to a patient if health care providers such as home health agencies were utilized. These alternatives are not always available in all communities and even where they exist they may not be available when needed.

EXAMPLE: Where the residents of a rural community generally utilize the outpatient facilities of a hospital located some distance from the area, the hospital outpatient department constitutes an alternative source of care that is available to the community. Roads in winter, however, may be impassable for some periods of time and in special situations institutionalization might be needed.

In determining the availability of more economical care alternatives, the coverage or noncoverage of that alternative care is not a factor to be considered. Home health care for a patient who is not homebound, for example, may be an appropriate alternative in some cases. The fact that such care cannot be covered by Medicare is irrelevant.

The issue is feasibility and not whether coverage is provided in one setting and not provided in another. For instance, an individual in need of daily skilled physical therapy might be able to receive the services needed on a more economical basis from an independently practicing physical therapist. However, the fact that Medicare reimbursement could not be made for the services because the $500 expense limitation applicable to the services of an independent physical therapist had been exceeded or because the patient was not enrolled in Part B, would not be a basis for determining that, as a practical matter, the needed care could only be provided in a SNF.

In determining the availability of alternate facilities or services, whether the patient or another resource can pay for the alternate services is not a factor to be considered.

> AVAILABILITY MEANS THAT A USUALLY LESS COSTLY ALTERNATIVE ACTUALLY EXISTS AND THAT, IN THEORY, IT COULD BE USED.

B. *Whether Available Alternatives are More Economical in the Individual Case.*—If you determine that a generally more economical care alternative is available to provide the needed care, consider whether the use of the alternative actually would be more economical in the individual case.

EXAMPLE: If a patient's condition requires daily transportation to the alternative source of care (e.g., a hospital outpatient department) by ambulance, it might be more economical from a health care delivery viewpoint to provide the needed care in the SNF setting.

EXAMPLE: If needed care could be provided in the home, but the patient's residence is so isolated that daily visits would entail inordinate travel costs, care in an SNF might be a more economical alternative.

ECONOMY IN THE INDIVIDUAL CASE IS MEASURED WITHOUT REGARD TO WHICH PARTIES BEAR WHAT SHARE OF THE COST. AN ALTERNATIVE MAY BE CHEAPER FOR MEDICARE BUT NOT BE MORE ECONOMICAL BECAUSE THE TOTAL COST OF USING IT WOULD EQUAL OR EXCEED THE COST OF SNF CARE.

C. *Whether the Patient's Physical Condition Would Permit Him to Utilize an Available, More Economical Care Alternative.*—In determining the practicality of using more economical care alternatives, consider the patient's medical condition. If the use of those alternatives would adversely affect the patient's medical condition, conclude that as a practical matter the daily skilled services can only be provided by an SNF on an inpatient basis.

If the use of a care alternative involves transportation of the individual on a daily basis, consider whether daily transportation would cause excessive physical hardship. Determinations on whether a patient's condition would be adversely affected if an available, more economical care alternative were utilized should not be based solely on the fact that the patient is nonambulatory. There are individuals confined to wheelchairs who, though nonambulatory, could be transported daily by automobile from their homes to alternative care sources without any adverse impact. Conversely, there are instances where an individual's condition would be adversely affected by daily transportation to a care facility, even though he is able to ambulate to some extent.

EXAMPLE: A 75-year-old woman has suffered a cerebrovascular accident and cannot climb stairs with safety. The patient lives alone in a second-floor apartment accessible only by climbing a flight of stairs. She requires physical therapy and occupational therapy on alternate days, and they are only available in a CORF one mile away from her apartment. However, because of her inability to negotiate the stairs, the daily skilled services she requires cannot, as a practical matter, be provided to the patient outside the SNF.

FINALLY, IF THERE IS AN ALTERNATIVE THAT IS BOTH AVAILABLE AND MORE ECONOMICAL, IT ALSO MUST BE FEASIBLE FOR THE PARTICULAR PATIENT.

The "practical matter" criterion should never be interpreted so strictly that it results in the automatic denial of coverage for patients who have been meeting all of the SNF level of care requirements, but who have occasion to be away from the SNF for a brief period of time. While most beneficiaries requiring an SNF level of care find that they are unable to leave the facility for even the briefest of time, the fact that a patient is granted an outside pass, or short leave of absence, for the purpose of attending a special religious service, holiday meal or family occasion, is not by itself evidence that the individual no longer needs to be in a SNF for his or her required skilled care. Very often special arrangements, not feasible on a daily basis, have had to be made to allow the absence from the facility. Where frequent or prolonged periods away from the SNF become possible, however, then questions as to whether the patient's care can, as a practical matter, only be furnished on an inpatient basis in an SNF may be raised. Decisions in these cases should be based on information reflecting the care needed and received by the patient while in the SNF and on the arrangements needed for the provision, if any, of this care during any absences. (See §3135.3 for counting inpatient days during a leave of absence.)

A conservative approach to retain the presumption for waiver of liability may lead a facility to notify patients that leaving the facility will result in denial of coverage. Such a notice is not appropriate. If an SNF determines that covered care is no longer needed, the situation does not change whether the patient actually leaves the facility or not. (See §3439.2, *Improper Provider Coverage Decisions*.)

THIS MATERIAL IS UNCHANGED FROM THE PREVIOUS INSTRUCTION. CAREFUL JUDGMENT IS NEEDED TO DECIDE IF A LEAVE OF ABSENCE RAISES THE ISSUE OF "PRACTICAL MATTER."

END OF MANUAL GUIDELINES

REHABILITATION: PATIENT'S POTENTIAL FOR RECOVERY

Several readers believe that the new guidelines make conflicting statements about the influence that a patient's potential for recovery should have on coverage of rehabilitation.

Let us explore this in detail and see if such conflicts exist. First, we should emphasize that these guidelines, like all HCFA guidelines, must be read *in entirety*. Phrases cannot be lifted out of them, removed from context, and portrayed as universal rules.

There has been an unfortunate tendency on the part of some readers to scan through the 14 pages of text and try to extract a few sentences as the "real" rules. The rest of the material is then disregarded as irrelevant. This practice can only promote misunderstanding.

Section 3132.1.B., page 3–56.14, makes three statements on this issue:

- While a patient's condition is a factor in deciding if skilled services *are* needed, it should never be the sole factor in deciding that a service is *not* skilled.
- The deciding factor in determining if rehabilitation services are skilled is whether the skills of a therapist are needed, not the patient's potential for recovery.
- A usually nonskilled service can, because of complications, require the skills of a therapist.

This last principle must not be overlooked. In special cases the ordinary view of a service as nonskilled can be overturned because of the patient's condition. This means that a service that ordinarily is considered nonskilled, under the general requirements for skilled therapy, can be treated as a skilled service in these special cases.

Those general requirements for skilled physical therapy are presented in section 3132.3.A.1, on pages 3–56.19-20. Two requirements that pertain to this issue are

- The level of the services, *or* the condition of the patient, must require the skills of a physical therapist.
- There must be a reasonable expectation of improvement in the patient's condition, *or* the services must be needed to establish a maintenance program.

Section 3132.3.A.2, pages 3–56.20-21, goes on to discuss specific physical therapy modalities:

- Therapeutic exercises can be skilled due either to the type of exercise *or* to the patient's condition.
- Repetitive maintenance exercises *sometimes might* require the skills of a therapist because of the level of the procedures used. (Cross-reference is made to 3132.1.B.)
- Heat treatments *might* require the skills of a therapist, due to complications in the patient's condition.

Section 3132.4, pages 3–57.1+2, identifies certain nonskilled services but also says they could be skilled if the circumstances in 3132.1.B. are met. Repetitive maintenance exercises are identified as nonskilled *if* the skills of a therapist are not needed.

Reading all of these sections in context leads to a logical conclusion. If you determine that there is not a reasonable expectation of improvement in a patient's condition, you still do not know conclusively that skilled therapy is not needed. There may be a need for skilled services to establish a maintenance program. Or a special medical complication might require skilled services to perform exercises or treatments that normally are considered nonskilled.

We believe this analysis shows the so-called conflicts are not real, but stem from extracting statements out of context.

APPROPRIATENESS OF ADMISSION TO SNF

There is still a requirement for a prior hospital stay to qualify for SNF coverage. That requirement is discussed in sections 3131-3131.3 of the Intermediary Manual. It is separate from the level of care requirements.

Some of the examples used in the level of care guidelines have been questioned in terms of whether they might represent premature hospital discharges. All of the examples are intended *only* to illustrate whether the SNF care can be covered.

What happened to the patient before entering the SNF, and whether transfer to the SNF raises questions about the appropriateness of the hospital's actions, are outside the scope of these guidelines. None of the examples are meant to condone premature discharge from a hospital.

Part **III**

SUGGESTIONS FOR THE HEALTH CARE PROFESSIONAL

A Practical Guide
for Helping the Client

SUGGESTIONS FOR THE HEALTH CARE PROFESSIONAL

Diagnosis

1. In suspected cases of dementia, the importance of the case history cannot be overemphasized.
2. Whenever possible, the case history should be taken from someone close to the client.
3. Look for the following language signs: good syntax, poor content, poor engagement, difficulty in defining, difficulty in writing to dictation, empty speech, difficulty in staying with the topic.
4. Many dementia clients deny the existence of a problem. If this is the case, do not insist that the client recognize his or her shortcomings.

Treatment

1. Be realistic. Don't hope for the impossible. If you expect to alter the course or outcome of the disease, your therapy will be misdirected.
2. Develop a plan of action and new strategies based on the client's current function and need.
3. Do not work alone. Include significant others in your plan. Ongoing reinforcement is the key to successful therapy.
4. Remember, the overall goal is improved functional communication skills between the client and significant others. Therapy should be carried out within the context in which it will be used.
5. Identify your client's needs and the steps required to fulfill those needs.
6. Identify all the barriers to successful treatment.
7. Address the client directly and by name.
8. Always identify yourself by name.

9. Establish eye contact with the client before attempting to communicate.
10. Allow sufficient time for the client to respond.
11. Repeat often.
12. Do not offer choices unless you are certain that the client can choose.
13. Keep directions short, simple, and to the point.
14. Since therapy has a limited time span, train the significant other to continue working with the client after treatment is terminated.
15. Clients must be evaluated periodically after discharge, and, if necessary, treatment strategies should be modified.

HELPFUL HINTS FOR THE FAMILY

The following suggestions are addressed to caregivers of dementia clients.

1. The secret of success in handling the dementia client can be stated in one word: consistency. Whatever you do, always do it the same way and, if possible, at the same time.
2. Any change in the client's performance should be noted. It may just be a bad day; however, if the behavior change persists for three or more days in a row, the client needs to be evaluated.
3. Sainthood is not a requirement. When things do not go well, anger and distress on the part of the client and yourself are normal and acceptable.
4. If the client wears dentures, be certain to check their fit. The dementia client may not be able to let you know if they are loose or rubbing.
5. A dementia client may not be able to wait to find a bathroom once he or she has left home. The following three steps can ease this problem.

   - Do not leave home without having the client use the bathroom.
   - When you arrive at your destination, locate the nearest bathroom.
   - If it has been more than two hours since the client has used the bathroom, ask if he or she needs to do so. If the client's responses are not reliable, do not ask but take the client to the bathroom and say, "I think it would be a good idea if you used the bathroom now." Do not wait for the client to ask to use the bathroom.

6. It is a good idea to carry a plastic bag with a change of clothing. If the client is occasionally incontinent, it is better to be prepared than to worry about what to do later.
7. Panty hose are difficult for dementia clients to handle. Try ladies' kneehighs or socks.
8. Low-heeled or flat crepe-soled shoes help the unsteady client.
9. The client should wear an identification bracelet that lists his or her name, address, telephone number, and the fact that he or she has a disease that causes confusion and an inability to relay accurate information. A simple statement such as "memory loss" may be sufficient.
10. For a successful shopping trip:

    - pick a place that is accessible.
    - try to do all your shopping in one store.
    - shop only when the store is not crowded.
    - make a map of the store and identify the location of items that you plan to purchase.

- list the items that you plan to purchase according to the route you will take in the store. The objective is to have all the items in the cart after your first walk through the store.
- have the client push the cart (this helps to prevent wandering).

11. When choosing photographs of family and friends for identification purposes, be certain to use the latest picture. An old photograph can be confusing.
12. Information regarding appointments or trips should not be given to the client more than one day in advance to prevent irritability.
13. Do not try to reason with someone who by definition is unreasonable.
14. Acknowledge when the client is confused, then orient him or her.
15. Lighting is important in maintaining good orientation. Twinkling lights, a dim atmosphere, reflecting mirrored lights, or candlelight can confuse the dementia client.
16. If you would like to have a meal out but the client has difficulty with eating utensils, order finger food (for example, a sandwich and french fries).
17. You do not have to shout to make yourself understood. Frequent repetition using simple sentences coupled with good eye contact will do a better job.
18. Review the environment that the client lives in. Steps may be a hazard and require gates; sharp objects and poisonous substances should be out of reach.

ADDITIONAL SOURCES OF INFORMATION ABOUT ALZHEIMER'S DISEASE AND AGING

Alzheimer's Disease and Related Disorders Association, Inc. (ADRDA)
919 North Michigan Avenue
Chicago, IL 60611
312/335-8700

Alzheimer's Disease Education and Referral Center (ADEAR)
(A service of the National Institute on Aging, NIH)
Address: ADEAR Center
PO Box 8250
Silver Spring, MD 20907-8250
Telephone: 800/438-4380
Fax: 301/495-3334
Internet: www.alzheimers.org
E-mail: adear@alzheimers.org

American Association of Retired Persons (AARP)
601 E Street NW
Washington, DC 20049
800/424-3410
202/434-2277
Internet: www.aarp.org

American Occupational Therapy Association (AOTA)
4720 Montgomery Lane
PO Box 31220
Bethesda, MD 20824-1220
800/729-2682

American Physical Therapy Association
1111 North Fairfax Street
Alexandria, VA 22314
800/999-2782

Gerontological Society of America
1275 K Street NW, Suite 350
Washington, DC 20005-4006
202/842-1275

National Council of Senior Citizens
1331 F Street NW
Washington, DC 20004
202/347-8800 or 202/624-9500

National Institute on Aging
National Institutes of Health
Bethesda, MD 20892
301/496-4400
Internet: www.nih.gov/nia

National Association of Social Workers
750 1st Street NE, Suite 700
Washington, DC 20002
202/408-8600

Bibliography

Adams, R.D., & Victor, M. (1977). *Principles of neurology* (3rd ed.). New York: McGraw-Hill.

Albert, M.L., Goodglass, H., Helm, M.A., Reubens, A.B., & Alexander, M.P. (1981). *Clinical aspects of dysphasia.* New York: Springer-Verlag.

Alfrey, Le Gendre, G.R., & Kaehny, W.D. (1976). The dialysis encephalopathy syndrome. Possible aluminum intoxication. *New England Journal of Medicine, 4,* 184–188.

Alzheimer, A. (1907). Uber eine eigen artige Erkrankung der Hirnrindle. *Allg Zeit Psychiatrie und PsychischGrichtlich Medicin, 64,* 146.

American Psychiatric Association. (1980). *Diagnostic and Statistical Manual of Mental Disorders* (3rd ed.). Washington, DC: author.

Appell, J., Kertesz, A., & Fisman, M. (1982). A study of language functioning in Alzheimer clients. *Brain & Language, 17,* 73–91.

Ashford, J.W., Kolm, P., Colliver, J.A., Bekian, C., & Hsu, L. (1989). Alzheimer Patient Evaluation and the Mini-Mental State: Item Characteristic Curve Analysis. *Journal of Gerontology: Psychological Sciences, 44*(5), 139–146.

Banner, C. (1992). Recent insights into the biology of Alzheimer's disease. *Generations Journal of the American Society on Aging, 16*(4), 31–34.

Barker, M.G., & Lawson, J.S. (1968). Nominal aphasia in dementia. *British Journal of Psychiatry, 114,* 1351–1356.

Bartol, M.A. (1979). Nonverbal communication in patients with Alzheimer's disease. *Journal of Gerontological Nursing, 5,* 21–31.

Bayles, K.A., & Boone, D.R. (1979, November). *Language and speech in normal senescence and senility.* Paper presented at the American Speech-Language-Hearing Association, Atlanta, Georgia.

Bayles, K.A., & Boone, D.R. (1982). The potential of language tasks for identifying senile dementia. *Journal of Speech and Hearing Disorders, 47,* 21–217.

Bayles, K.A., & Kaszniak, A.W. (1991). *Communication and cognition in normal aging and dementia.* Austin, TX: Pro. ed.

Beasley, D.S., & Davis, G.A. (1981). *Aging: Communication processes and disorders.* New York: Grune & Stratton.

Besdine, R.W. (1983). The educational utility of comprehensive functional assessment in the elderly. *Journal of the American Geriatrics Society, 31,* 651–656.

Boller, F., Mizutani, T., Roessman, U., & Gambetti, P.L. (1980). Parkinson's disease, dementia and Alzheimer's disease: Clinico-pathological correlations. *Annals of Neurology, 7,* 329–335.

Bollinger, R. & Hardiman, C.J. (1991). *Rating scale of communication in cognitive decline* (1st ed.). Buffalo, N.Y: United Educational Services.

Bouchard, M.M., & Shane, H.C. (1977). Use of the problem-oriented medical record in the speech and hearing profession. *ASHA, 19,* 157–159.

Bowen, D.M., Smith, C.B., White, P., & Davidson, A.N. (1979). Neurotransmitter-related enzymes and indices of hypoxia in senile dementia and other abiotrophies. *Brain, 99,* 459–496.

Brody, S.J., & Ruff, G.E. (Eds.). (1986). *Aging and rehabilitation.* New York: Springer.

Brun, A. (1983). An overview of light and electron microscopic changes. In B. Reisberg (Ed.), *Alzheimer's disease: The standard reference* (pp. 37–45). New York: The Free Press.

Butters, N., & Cermak, L.W. (1980). *Alcoholic Korsakoff's syndrome: An information-processing approach to America.* New York: Academic Press.

Cairl, R.E., Pfeiffer, E., Keller, D.M., Burke, H., & Samis, H.V. (1983). An evaluation of the reliability and validity of the Functional Assessment Inventory. *Journal of the American Geriatrics Society, 31,* 607–612.

Chartier-Harlin, M.C., et al. (1991). Early-onset Alzheimer's disease caused by mutations at codon 717 of the beta-amyloid precursor protein gene. *Nature, 353,* 844–846.

Comptroller General of the United States. (1979). *Conditions of older people: National information systems needed* (U.S. General Accounting Office Publication No. HRD–79–75). Washington, DC: Government Printing Office.

Corkin, S. (1982). Some relationships between global amnesia and the memory impairments in Alzheimer's disease. In S. Corkin, K.L. Davis, J.H. Growdon, E. Usdin, & R.J. Wurtman (Eds.), *Alzheimer's disease: A report of progress in research* (pp. 149–164). New York: Raven.

Corkin, S., Growdon, J.H., Sullivan, E.V., & Shedlack, K. (1981, February). Lecithin and cognitive function in aging and dementia. In A.D. Kidman, J.K. Tomkins, R.A. Westerman (Eds.), *Proceedings of the Second Symposium of the Foundation for Life Sciences* (pp. 229–247). Sydney, Australia.

Crapper, D.R., & Dalton, A.J. (1973). Alteration in short-term retention, conditioned avoidance, acquisition, and motivation following aluminum-induced neurofibrillary degeneration. *Physiology & Behavior, 10,* 925–933.

Crapper, D.R., Harlik, S., de Boni, U. (1978). Aluminum and other metals in senile (Alzheimer) dementia. In R. Katzman, R.D. Terry, & K.L. Bick (Eds.), *Alzheimer's disease: Senile dementia and related disorders.* New York: Raven.

Crapper, D.R., Krishman, S.S., & Dalton, A.J. (1973). Brain aluminum distribution in Alzheimer's disease and experimental neurofibrillary degeneration. *Science, 180,* 511–513.

Crystal, H.A., Horoupian, D.S., Katzman, R., & Jotkowitz, S. (1982). Biopsy-proved Alzheimer's disease presenting as a right parietal lobe syndrome. *Annals of Neurology, 12,* 186–188.

Cummings, J. (1984a). Dementia: Definition, classification, and differential diagnosis. *Psychiatric Annals, 14,* 85–89.

Cummings, J. (1984b, November). Dementia: A clinical approach. Short course presented at the American Speech-Language-Hearing Association Meetings, San Francisco, CA.

Cummings, J., Benson, D.F., Hill, M.A., & Read, S. (1985). Aphasia in dementia of the Alzheimer's type. *Neurology (New York), 35,* 394–396.

Davies, P., & Maloney, A.J. (1976). Selective loss of central cholinergic neurons in Alzheimer's disease. *Lancet, 2,* 1403.

Davis, C.M. (1986). The role of the physical and occupational therapist in caring for the victim of Alzheimer's disease. In E.D. Taira (Ed.), *Therapeutic interventions for the person with dementia* (pp. 15–28). New York: The Haworth Press.

De Millano, M. (1984). Eight common charting mistakes to avoid. *Nursing Life, 4,* 30–32.

Dunkle, R.E. (1984). Differential diagnosis: The key to appropriate treatment. In C.R. Hooper & R.E. Dunkle (Eds.), *The Older Aphasic Person* (pp. 69–127). Rockville, MD: Aspen Publishers.

Ernst, B., Dalby, A., & Dalby, M.A. (1970a). Aphasic disturbances in presenile dementia. *Acta Neurologica Scandinavia (Suppl.), 43,* 99–100.

Ernst, B., Dalby, M.A., & Dalby, A. (1970b). Gnostic praxic disturbances in presenile dementia. *Acta Neurologica Scandinavia (Suppl.), 43,* 101–102.

Fillenbaum, G.U., & Smyer, M.A. (1981). The development, validity, and reliability of the OARS multidimensional functional assessment questionnaire. *Journal of Gerontology, 36,* 428–434.

Folstein, M.D., Folstein, S.E., & McHugh, P.R. (1975). Mini-Mental State: A practical method for grading the cognitive state of patients for the clinician. *Journal of Psychiatric Research, 12,* 189–198.

Fortinsky, M.A., Granger, C.V., & Seltzer, G.B. (1981). The use of functional assessment in understanding home care needs. *Medical Care, 29,* 489–497.

Fuld, P.A. (1983). Word intrusion as a diagnostic sign in Alzheimer's disease. *Geriatric Medicine Today, 2*(4).

Gajdusek, D.C., & Gibbs, C.J. (1964). Slow, latent and temperate virus infections of the central nervous system. *Research Publications of the Association for Research on Nervous and Mental Disorders, 44,* 254–280.

Gibbs, C.J., & Gajdusek, D.C. (1978). Subacute spongiform virus encephalopathies: The transmissible virus dementias. In R. Katzman, R.D. Terry, & K.L. Bick (Eds.), *Alzheimer's disease: Senile dementia and related disorders* (pp. 559–575). New York: Raven.

Gilbert, J.G., & Levee, R.F. (1971). Patterns of declining memory. *Journal of Gerontology, 26,* 70–75.

Glickstein, J.K., & Neustadt, G.K. (1995). *Reimbursable geriatric service delivery: A functional maintenance therapy system.* Gaithersburg, MD: Aspen Publishers.

Glickstein, J.K., & Raiff, N.R. (1985, October). Family members as evaluation specialists: Incorporating lay perspectives in functional assessment of the elderly. Paper presented at the Pennsylvania Sociological Society annual meeting, Pittsburgh, PA.

Goate, A. et al., (1991). Segregation of mis-sense mutation in the amyloid precursor protein gene with familial Alzheimer's disease. *Nature 349,* 704–706.

Goldgaber, D., Lerman, M.I., McBride, O.W., Safflotti, D., & Gajdusek, D.C. (1987). Characterization and chromosomal localization of a cDNA-encoding brain amyloid of Alzheimer's disease. *Science, 235,* 877–880.

Goodglass, H., & Kaplan, E. (1972). *Assessment of aphasia and related disorders.* Philadelphia: Lea and Febiger.

Granger, C., Dewis, L.S., Peters, N.C., Sherwood, C.C., & Barrett, J.E. (1979). Stroke rehabilitation: Analysis of repeated Barthel Index measures. *Archives of Physical Medicine and Rehabilitation, 60,* 14–17.

Grauer, H., & Birnbom, F. (1975). A geriatric functional rating scale to determine the need for institutional care. *Journal of the American Geriatrics Society, 23,* 472–476.

Gurland, B., Kuriansky, J., Sharpe, L., Simon, R., Stiller, P., & Birkett, P. (1978). The comprehensive assessment and referral evaluation (CARE)—rationale, development, and reliability. *International Journal of Aging and Human Development, 8*(1), 9–42.

Gwyther, L.P. (1985). *Care of Alzheimer's patients: A manual for nursing home staff.* New York: American Health Care Association and Alzheimer's Disease and Related Disorders Association.

Gwyther, L.P., & Matteson, M.A. (1983). Care for the caregivers. *Journal of Gerontological Nursing, 9*(2).

Haney, D.Q. (1996, March 21). Brain imagery exposes a killer. *Pittsburgh Post Gazette, 69*(234), 6.

Harris, L. (1981, November). *Aging in the fifties: America in transition.* Washington, DC: National Council on the Aging.

Health Care Finance Administration. (1982). *Developments in aging: 1982,* vol. 1. Washington, DC: U.S. Senate Special Committee on Aging.

Health Care Finance Administration. (1995). *Resident Assessment Instrument: MDS Version 2.0.* State Operations Manual. Washington, D.C.: U.S. Department of Health and Human Services.

Heilman, K.M. (1979). Apraxia. In K.M. Heilman & E. Valenstein (Eds.), *Clinical neuropsychology* (pp. 159–185). New York: Oxford University Press.

Heston, L.L. (1977). Alzheimer's disease, trisomy 21, and myeloproliferative disorders: Associations suggesting a genetic diathesis. *Science, 196,* 322–323.

Heston, L.L. (1979). Alzheimer's disease and senile dementia: Genetic relationships to Down syndrome and hematologic cancer. *Research Publications of the Association for Research in Nervous and Mental Disease, 57,* 167–176.

Heston, L.L., & Mastri, A. (1977). The genetics of Alzheimer's Disease—Associations with hematologic malignancy and Down Syndrome. *Archives of General Psychiatry, 34,* 976–981.

Heston, L.L., & White, J. (1978). Pedigrees of 30 families with Alzheimer's disease: Association with defective organization of microfilaments and microtubules. *Behavioral Genetics, 8,* 315–331.

Hoyert, D.L. (1993, November). Increases in Alzheimer's as a cause-of-death. Paper presented at the annual meeting of the Gerontological Society of America, New Orleans, LA.

Hughes, J.R., & Cayaffa, J.J. (1977). The EEG in patients at different ages without organic cerebral disease. *Electroencephalography and Clinical Neurophysiology, 42,* 776–784.

Hutchinson, T.A., Boyd N.F., & Feinstein, A.R. (1979). Scientific problems in clinical scales as demonstrated in the Karnofsky Index of Performance status. *Journal of Chronic Diseases, 32,* 661–666.

Katz, S., Ford, A B., Moskowitz, R.W., Jackson, B.A., & Jaffe, M.W. (1963). Studies of illness in the aged: The index of ADL, a standardized measure of biological and psychosocial function. *Journal of the American Medical Association, 185,* 914–919.

Katzman, R., Terry, R.D., & Bick, K.L. (1978). Recommendations of the nosology, epidemiology, and etiology and pathophysiology commissions of the workshop-conference on Alzheimer's disease. Senile dementia and related disorders. In R. Katzman, R.D. Terry, & K.L. Bick (Eds.), *Alzheimer's disease: Senile dementia and related disorders.* New York: Raven.

Kim, Y., Morrow, L., & Boller, F. (1980). Patterns of intellectual impairment in Alzheimer's and Huntington's diseases. *International Neurological Society Bulletin, 3,* 20–21.

Kirshner, H.S., Webb, W.G., Kelly, M.P., & Wells, C.E. (1984). Language disturbance: An initial symptom of cortical degeneration and dementia. *Archives of Neurology, 41,* 491–496.

Klatzo, I., Wisniewski, H., & Streicher, E. (1965). Experimental production of neurofibrillary degeneration. *Journal of Neuropathology and Experimental Neurology, 24,* 187–199.

Koitz, D., Reuter, J., and Merlis, M. (1989, March 1). Medicare: Its use, funding, and economic dimensions. *CRS Report for Congress.* Washington, D.C.: Congressional Research Service, Library of Congress.

Krauss, I.C. (1962). Use of a comprehensive rating scale system in the institutional care of geriatric patients. *Journal of the American Geriatrics Society, 10,* 95–102.

Lawton, M.P., & Brody, E.M. (1969). Assessment of older people: Self-maintaining and instrumental activities of daily living. *The Gerontologist, 9,* 180–186.

Lee, V.M.-Y. et al. (1991). A68: A major subunit of paired helical filaments and derivatized forms of normal tau. *Science, 251,* 675–678.

Lewis, C.E., & Deigh, R.A. (1973). Project SIC: A survey of innovative changes in health care. *UCLA Center for Health Sciences Progress Report, 4,* 1–4.

Lipowski, Z.J. (1981). Organic mental disorders: Their history and classification with special reference to DSM-III. *Aging (New York), 15,* 37–45.

Mace, N. (1984, Fall). Report of a survey of day care centers. *Pride Institute Journal of Long-Term Home Care, 3*(4), 38–43.

Mace, N., & Rabins, P.V. (1981). *The Thirty-Six Hour Day.* Baltimore: The Johns Hopkins University Press.

Maddox, G.L. (1972). Intervention and outcomes: Notes on designing and implementing an experiment in health care. *International Journal of Epidemiology, 1,* 339–345.

Mager, R.F. (1984). *Preparing Instructional Objectives* (Rev. 2nd ed.). Belmont, CA: Robert F. Pitman Learning.

Mahoney, F.S., & Barthel, D.W. (1965). Functional evaluation: The Barthel Index. *Maryland State Medical Journal, 14,* 61–68.

Mahurin, R.K., DeBettinges B.H., & Pirozzolo F.J. (1996). Structured assessment of independent living skills: Preliminary report of a performance measure of functional abilities in dementia. *Topics in Geriatric Rehabilitation, 11*(4), 70–73.

Mathew, R.J., Meyer, J.S., Francis, D.J., Semchuk, K.M., Mortel, K., & Claghorn, J.L. (1980). Cerebral blood flow in depression. *American Journal of Psychiatry, 137,* 1449–1450.

McDermott, J.R., Smith, A.I., Khalid, I., & Wisniewski, H.M. (1979). Brain aluminum in aging and Alzheimer's disease. *Neurology, 29,* 809–814.

McEvoy, C., & Patterson, R. (1986) . Behavioral treatment of deficit skills in dementia patients. *The Gerontologist, 26,* 475–478.

McKhann, G., Drachman, D., Folstein, M., Katzman, R., Price, D., & Stedlan, E.M. (1984). Clinical diagnosis of Alzheimer's disease: Report of the NINCDS-ADRDA work group under the auspices of the Department of Health and Human Services Task Force on Alzheimer's Disease. *Neurology, 34,* 939–943.

Mentis, M., Briggs-Whittaker, J., & Gramigna, G.D. (1995, October). Discourse topic management in senile dementia of the Alzheimer's type. *Journal of Speech and Hearing Research, 38,* 1054–1066.

Miller, E. (1981). The nature of the cognitive deficit in senile dementia. In N.E. Miller & G.D. Cohen (Eds.), *Clinical aspects of Alzheimer's disease and senile dementia* (pp. 103–120). New York: Raven.

Miller, G. (1983). Case management: The essential service. In C.J. Sanborn (Ed.), *Case Management in Mental Health Services* (pp. 3–13). New York: The Haworth Press.

Miller, N.E., & Cohen, G.D. (1981). Clinical aspects of Alzheimer's disease and senile dementia: Synopsis and future perspectives in assessment, treatment, and service delivery. In N.E. Miller & G.D. Cohen (Eds.), *Clinical aspects of Alzheimer's disease and senile dementia* (pp. 17–35). New York: Raven.

Morris, J.N., Sherwood, S., & Mor, V. (1984). An assessment tool for use in identifying functionally vulnerable persons in the community. *The Gerontologist, 24,* 373–379.

Morscheck, P. (1984, Fall). An overview of Alzheimer's disease and long-term care. *Pride Journal of Long-Term Health Care, 3*(4), 4–10.

Mortimer, J.A. (1980). Epidemiological aspects of Alzheimer's disease. In F.J. Pirozzolo & G.S. Mali (Eds.), *The aging nervous system* (pp. 307–332). New York: Praeger.

Murrell, J. et al. (1991). A mutation in the amyloid precursor protein associated with hereditary Alzheimer's disease. *Science, 254,* 97–99.

Naeser, M.A., Gebhardt, M.A., & Levine, H.L. (1980). Decreased computerized tomography numbers in patients with presenile dementia. *Archives of Neurology, 37,* 401–409.

Nandy, K. (1978). Brain-reactive antibodies in aging and senile dementia. In R. Katzman, R.D. Terry, & K.L. Bick (Eds.), *Alzheimer's disease: Senile dementia and related disorders* (pp. 503–512). New York: Raven.

Nandy, K. (1983). Immunologic factors. In B. Reisberg (Ed.), *Alzheimer's disease: The standard reference* (pp. 135–138). New York: The Free Press.

Nissen, M.J., Corkin, S., Buonanno, F.S., Growdon, J.H., Wray, S.H., & Bauer, J. (1985). Spatial vision in Alzheimer's disease: General findings and a case report. *Archives of Neurology, 42,* 667–688.

Obler, L. (1979). Psycholinguistic aspects of language in dementia. Paper presented at the symposium on Language and Communication in Healthy and Dementing Elderly, Academy of Aphasia, San Diego, CA.

Obler, L. (1983). Language and brain dysfunction in dementia. In S. Segalowitz (Ed.), *Language functions and brain organization* (pp. 267–282). New York: Academic Press.

Obler, L. (1985, November). Language in aging and dementia. Short course presented at the American Speech-Language-Hearing Association Meetings, Washington, DC.

Obler, L.K., & Albert, M.I. (1981). Language and aging: A neurobehavioral analysis. In D. Beasley & G. Davis (Eds.), *Aging: Communication processes and disorders.* New York: Grune and Stratton.

Omnibus Budget Reconciliation Act of 1987, pub.l. no. 100-203, 101 Stat. 1330 (codified at 42 U.S.C.A.§1396 (Supp. 189). Also see 54 Fed. Reg. 5359-73 (codified at 42 C.F.R. Part 483, Subpart B).

Paulson, G.W. (1977). The neurological examination in dementia. In C.E. Wells (Ed.), *Dementia* (pp. 169–188). Philadelphia: Davis.

Physicians Desk Reference. (1996). Montvale, NJ: Medical Economics.

Perry, E.K., Perry, R.H., Blessed, G., & Tomlinson, B.E. (1977). Necropsy evidence of central cholinergic deficits in senile dementia. *Lancet, 3,* 1891.

Perry, E.K., Tomlinson, B.E., Blessed, G., Bergman, K., Gibson, P.H., & Perry, R.H. (1978). Correlation of cholinergic abnormalities with senile plaques and mental test scores in senile dementia. *British Medical Journal, 2,* 1457–1459.

Pfeiffer, E. (1975). A short portable mental status questionnaire for the assessment of organic brain deficit in elderly patients. *Journal of the American Geriatrics Society, 23,* 433–441.

The President's Commission on Mental Health. (1978). *Report to the President, Vol. 1.* Washington, DC: U.S. Department of Health, Education, and Welfare, Federal Council on Aging, U.S. Government Printing Office.

Rabins, P.V. (1984). Management of dementia in the family context. *Psychosomatics, 24,* 369–374.

Recer, Paul (1996, May 14) Test aims at Alzheimer's detection. *Pittsburgh Post-Gazette, 69* (288), A-2.

Reisberg, B. (Ed.). (1983). *Alzheimer's disease: The standard reference.* New York: The Free Press.

Reisberg, B. (1984). Stages of cognitive decline. *American Journal of Nursing, 84,* 225–228.

Reisberg, B., Ferris, S.H., & Crook, T. (1983). The Global Deterioration Scale (GDS) for Age-Associated Cognitive and Alzheimer's Disease. In B. Reisberg (Ed.), *Alzheimer's disease: The standard reference* (pp. 174–175). New York: The Free Press.

Rochford, G. (1971). A study of naming errors in dysphasic and in demented patients. *Neuropsychologia, 9,* 437–443.

Ross, M., Riffer, N., & Switalski, T. (1983). The experience in New York State. In C.J. Sanborn (Ed.), *Case Management in Mental Health Services* (pp. 101–112). New York: The Haworth Press.

Rubenstein, L.Z., Schairer, C., Weiland, G.D., & Kane, R. (1984). Systematic biases in functional status assessment of elderly adults: Effects of different data sources. *Journal of Gerontology, 39,* 686–691.

Sanders, H.I., & Warrington, E.K. (1971). Memory for remote events in amnesic patients. *Brain, 94,* 661–668.

Sarno, M.T. (1969). The functional communication profile manual of directions. *Rehabilitation Monograph, 42.*

Schneck, M.K., Reisberg, B., & Ferris, S.H. (1982). An overview of current concepts of Alzheimer's disease. *American Journal of Psychiatry, 139,* 165–173.

Schwartz, M., Martin, O.S.M., & Saffran, E.M. (1979). Disassociations of language functions in dementia: A case study. *Brain and Language, 7,* 177–306.

Selkoe, D.J., Bell, D., Podlisny, M.B., Price, D.L., & Cork, L.C. (1987). Conservation of brain amyloid proteins in aged mammals and humans with Alzheimer's disease. *Science, 235,* 873–876.

Sigurdsson, B. (1954). Rida, a chronic encephalitis of sheep with general remarks on infections which develop slowly and some of their special characteristics. *British Veterinary Journal, 110,* 341–343.

Sjogren, H. (1952). Clinical analysis of morbus Alzheimer and morbus Pick. *Acta Psychiatrica et Neurologica Scandanavia (Suppl.), 82,* 68–115.

St. George-Hyslop, P.H. (1987). The genetic defect causing familial Alzheimer's disease maps on chromosome 21. *Science, 235,* 885–890.

Stam, F.C., & Op Den Velde, W. (1978). Haptoglobin types in Alzheimer's disease and senile dementia. In R. Katzman, R.D. Terry, & K.L. Bick (Eds.), *Alzheimer's disease: Senile dementia and related disorders.* New York: Raven Press.

Steinberg, R.M. (1985). Access assistance and case management. In A. Monk (Ed.), *Handbook of Gerontological Services.* New York: Van Nostrand Reinhold.

Tanzi, R.E., Gusella, J.F., Watkins, P.C., Bruns, G.A.P., St. George-Hyslop, P., Van Keuren, M.L., Patterson. D., Pagan, S., Kurnit, D.M., & Neve, R.L. (1987). Amyloid β protein gene: cDNA, mRNA distribution, and genetic linkage near the Alzheimer locus. *Science, 235,* 880–884.

Tomlinson, B.E., Blessed, G., & Roth, M. (1970). Observations on the brains of demented old people. *Journal of Neurological Science, 11,* 205–242.

Trapp, G.A., Miner, G.D., & Zimmerman, R.L. (1978). Aluminum levels in brain in Alzheimer's disease. *BioPsychiatry, 13,* 709–718.

U.S. Bureau of the Census. (1982, October). *Decennial census of the population of the United States: 1982 to 2050 (advance report).* Current Population Reports, series P-25, No. 922. Washington, DC: U.S. Government Printing Office.

U.S. Department of Health and Human Services, Social Security Administration (Revised September 1986). *Income and Resources of the Population 65 and Over,* [SSA Publication no. 13-11727].

U.S. Department of Health and Human Services (1995, April). *Vital and Health Statistics: Trends in the Health of Older Americans: United States, 1994* [Publication No. (PHS) 95-1414] Series 3, No. 30 4-1988.

U.S. Department of Health and Human Services (1996, January). *Vital and Health Statistics: Mortality Trends for Alzheimer's Disease, 1979-91.* [Publication No. (PHS) 96-1856] Series 20: Data from the National Vital Statistics System No. 28. Hyattsville, MD: Centers for Disease Control and Prevention National Center for Health Statistics.

U.S. Senate Special Committee on Aging. (1983). *America in transition: An aging society, 1982* (vol. 1). Washington, DC: National Institute on Aging.

U.S. Senate Special Committee on Aging in conjunction with the American Association of Retired Persons. (1984). *Aging America: Trends and projections* [Publication No. PL3377 (584)]. Washington, DC: National Institute on Aging.

U.S. Senate Special Committee on Aging in conjunction with the American Association of Retired Persons. (1991). *Aging America: Trends and projections* [Publication No. LR3377 (991)]. Washington, DC: National Institute on Aging.

Wasow, M. (1986). Support groups for family caregivers of patients with Alzheimer's disease. *Social Work, 31*(2), 93–97.

Wechsler, A.F. (1977). Presenile dementia presenting as aphasia. *Journal of Neurology, Neurosurgery and Psychiatry, 40,* 303–305

Wechsler, D. (1958). *The measurement and appraisal of adult intelligence* (4th ed.). Baltimore: Williams and Wilkins.

White, P., Hiley, C.R., & Goodhardt, M.J. (1977). Neocortical cholinergic neurons in elderly people. *Lancet, 2,* 668–681.

Willanger, R., & Klee, A. (1966). Metamorphopsia and other visual disturbances with latency occurring in patients with diffuse cerebral lesions. *Acta Neurologica Scandinavia (Suppl.), 42,* 1–18.

Wurtman, R.J. (1985, January). Alzheimer's disease. *Scientific American, 252*(1), 62–74.

Yamaura, H., Masatoshi, I., Kubota, K., & Matsuzawa, T. (1980). Brain atrophy during aging: A quantitative study with computed tomography. *Journal of Gerontology, 35,* 492–498.

Glossary

Acetylcholine—a chemical compound necessary for the transmission of nerve impulses. This compound is severely reduced in the brains of Alzheimer's victims.

ADL—activities of daily living. Functions that are fundamental to independent living. These functions include bathing, dressing, toileting, transfer from bed or chair, continence, and feeding.

Agnosia—an acquired cortical sensory or perceptual disorder.

Alzheimer, Alois (1864–1915)—German physician who studied the relationship of changes in the nervous system to disease. He was the first to describe the neuropathological changes in Alzheimer's disease.

Alzheimer's disease (AD)—age-associated cognitive decline of gradual onset and course. Associated neuropathological changes are seen on autopsy.

Amyloid—a starch-like glycoprotein.

Aphasia—an acquired disorder of language due to brain injury.

Apolipoprotein E (APOE)—gene located on chromosome 19 that may be implicated in late onset Alzheimer's.

APP—amyloid precursor protein.

Apraxia—an impairment of voluntary movement, without obvious sensorimotor deficits.

Brain enzyme—a protein that accelerates a specific chemical reaction in the brain.

Choline—one of the elements needed for the body to manufacture acetylcholine. Choline is found in the vitamin B complex and is concentrated in foods such as eggs and meat.

Choline acetyltransferase (CAT)—an enzyme needed by the brain to stimulate the production of acetylcholine.

Chromosome—rodlike structures that carry the genes. Each animal species carries a set number of chromosomes that determine the make-up of the organism.

Chromosome 21—the particular chromosome that has been implicated in Alzheimer's disease and Down syndrome.

Creutzfeldt-Jakob disease—a rapidly progressive form of dementia caused by a slow-acting virus.

Dementia—a progressive form of mental impairment due to various underlying pathologic processes.

Dementia pugilistica—dementia seen in prize fighters that appears to progress in a manner similar to AD. Autopsied brains of persons with this type of dementia show the same type of tangles as those identified in AD.

DNA—deoxyribonucleic acid. A large molecule, shaped like a double helix and found primarily in the chromosomes of the cell nucleus, that contains the genetic information of the cell. The genetic information is coded in the sequence of subunits making up the DNA molecule.

Dopamine—the precursor of norepinephrine and epinephrine. It is present in the central nervous system and localized in the basal ganglia.

Gene—the unit of inheritance that is located on and transmitted by the chromosome and that develops into a hereditary character as it reacts with the environment and with other genes.

IADL—instrumental activities of daily living. Complex daily activities such as using the telephone or cooking a meal, that are essential fundamentals to independent living.

Kuru—an irreversible dementia caused by a slow-acting virus that occurs in some tribes in New Guinea.

Lymphoproliferative cancers—cancers of the lymphatic system such as Hodgkin's.

Metabolic disorder—a disturbance in the physical and chemical processes by which chemical compounds in the body are produced, maintained, and transformed into energy.

Multi-infarct dementia—the second most common type of dementia in older adults. It is attributed to multiple small infarcts or strokes and follows a step-wise course, with sudden onset and improvements noted. Many of the symptoms are similar to those of Alzheimer's disease.

Myoclonus—a rhythmical twitching of a muscle or group of muscles.

Neuritic plaques (senile plaques)—abnormal protein surrounded by bits of degenerated nerve fiber; the most conspicuous pathological changes found in people with AD. There are three distinct types of neuritic plaques: primitive, classical, and amyloid. In AD, primitive and classical plaques are particularly numerous in the cortex and the hippocampus. Amyloid plaques are generally limited to the cerebellar cortex.

Neurofibrillary tangle—abnormal fibers in the nerve cells of the cerebral cortex. The hallmark lesion of the Alzheimer brain. Also referred to as "Alzheimer neurofibrillary tangles" (NFTs) or "Alzheimer's neurofibrillary changes." They are composed of bundles of paired filaments: each filament of the pair is 10–13nm in diameter, helically wound around each other at regular intervals of 80nm.

Neurotransmitter—any specific chemical agent released by a presynaptic cell, upon excitation, which crosses the synapse to stimulate or inhibit the postsynaptic cell.

Noradrenaline (norepinephrine)—a chemical produced in the medulla of the adrenal gland which affects many physiological and metabolic activities.

Normal pressure hydrocephalus—a condition caused by increased fluid pressure within the ventricles of the brain. In addition to dementia, there are changes in gait and incontinence. A shunt is sometimes used to relieve the pressure.

Plaques—abnormal protein surrounded by bits of degenerated nerve fiber. Plaques are found at autopsy in the brains of individuals who had Alzheimer's disease.

Presenile dementia—a dementia syndrome with age of onset before age 65 including, but not limited to, Alzheimer's disease.

Protein—a chemical compound consisting of a long chain of amino acids, which contain a special grouping of nitrogen and hydrogen atoms. Protein may be obtained from the diet or produced by living cells.

Serotonin—a neurotransmitter; a vasoconstrictor, liberated by the blood platelets that inhibits gastric secretion and stimulates smooth muscle.

Scrapies—a progressive neurologic disorder that occurs in sheep, similar to "mad cow" disease.

Senile dementia—dementia syndrome with onset after age 65 due to an underlying pathology.

Somatostatin—a chemical capable of inhibiting the release of somatotropin (growth hormone) by the anterior lobe of the pituitary gland.

Tau protein—a normal component of nerve cells. When processed abnormally in AD Tau forms bundles of fibrous proteins composed in part of paired helical filaments or "tangles."

Materials

The following is a list of materials used in Unit 8, Lesson Plans:

1. Category Cards
   Contents:
   Blank labels, word labels, labels with pictures of objects. These labels are referred to in the text as "cards." They are used in lessons involving recall, memory, and reading.

   Peel-off labels and pictures

   a. Blank removable self-stick labels, $1'' \times 3''$
   b. Blank removable self-stick labels, $1\frac{1}{4}'' \times 1\frac{3}{4}''$
   c. Removable self-stick words, $1'' \times 3''$
   d. Removable self-stick pictures to match self-stick words, $1\frac{1}{4}'' \times 1\frac{3}{4}''$
   e. Matching removable self-stick action pictures, $2'' \times 2''$

2. Pencils that are easy to grasp because of their size or because of the addition of a special covering such as foam.

   a. Easy-grip pencil
   b. Chubby pencil

3. Magnetic Message Center (Reality Orientation Kit)
   Contents:
   Lightweight magnetic words, letters, and objects that can be attached to the client's refrigerator or any metal surface to serve as a reminder.
   a. Large magnetic board with stand or easel, $13'' \times 16''$, referred to as a magnetic Reality Board in text.

    b. Magnetic information words, 1″ × 6″
       Days of week
       Months of year
       Category words, 1″ × 6″ (food, clothing, household items, health aids)
    c. Magnetic clock
       Clock face (white with black trim), 10″ diameter
       Individual numbers (black or white), 1″ square
       Removable clock hands (black)
    d. Magnetic alphabet letters (all caps), 1″ × 1″
    e. Magnetic numbers 0 through 9, 1″ × 1″
    f. Wipe-off marker

4. Stand-up clock with moveable hands, 10″ diameter (this could be constructed from sturdy cardboard).

5. Picture pocket, 8″ × 10″ or 10″ × 10″
Clear 8″ × 10″ sheet of plastic that will hold four to six pictures and can be mounted on a wall with double-sided tape or on a metal surface with small magnets.

6. Small magnets (six)

7. Client/Reference List
This form is used when making lists and practicing. It is also used for documentation of work accomplished and of the client's progress (see Appendix D).

8. Simulated grocery items: a market basket with miniature grocery items.

How to Obtain Necessary Materials

Therapists have the option of purchasing or making their own materials. Simulated grocery items, wipe-off markers, and easy-grip pencils are available at most children's stores and places specializing in educational materials.

The following materials are needed to make the Category Cards.

1. $\frac{1}{2}'' \times 2''$ removable labels for word cards
2. $2'' \times 2''$ removable labels for picture cards
3. Pictures cut to fit $2'' \times 2''$ removable labels

Directions: Paste pictures on $2'' \times 2''$ removable labels. Type or print matching words on $\frac{1}{2}'' \times 2''$ removable labels. Removable labels are available at office supply stores. See Appendix D for a list of suggested words for "Basic Category Cards."

Enlarge the Client/Reference List at the end of Appendix D for use during the lesson.

Picture pockets may be purchased at any store selling photograph albums and can be mounted on a refrigerator or metal cabinet with four small magnets or on other surfaces with a thumbtack or tape.

Suggested Category Cards and Client/Reference List Form

FOOD

Bread
English muffins
Sweet rolls
Cake
Cookies
Salt
Pepper
Cereal
Coffee
Tea
Juice
Sugar
Jelly
Ice cream
TV dinners
Butter
Cheese
Yogurt
Milk
Eggs
Pickles

VEGETABLES

Peas
Corn
Carrots
Potatoes
Green beans
Beets
Celery
Lettuce
Tomatoes
Cucumbers
Onions

FRUITS

Apples
Bananas
Oranges
Grapefruit

MEAT

Roast beef
Chicken
Liver
Pork chops
Steak
Ground beef
Sausage
Bacon
Cold cuts
Fish

CLOTHING

Shorts
Underpants
Bra
Socks
Panty hose
Shoes
Pants
Belt
Shirt
Blouse
Skirt
Dress
Slip
Pajamas
Nightgown
Bathrobe
Slippers
Hat
Sweater
Coat
Raincoat
Rain boots
Mittens
Gloves
Umbrella
Scarf
Handkerchief

HOUSEHOLD NEEDS

Cleanser
Napkins
Soap
Detergent
Facial tissue
Toilet paper
Paper towels
Air freshener
Fabric softener
Bleach
Waxed paper
Aluminum foil
Plastic wrap
Laundry soap
Ammonia
Garbage bags
Glass cleaner

HEALTH AIDS

Nonaspirin pain reliever
Antacid
Eyeglasses
Hearing aid
Toothbrush
Toothpaste
Razor
Soap
Deodorant
Washcloth
Towel
Dentures
Hair brush
Comb
Lipstick
Powder
Shampoo
Mouthwash

CLIENT/REFERENCE LIST FORM

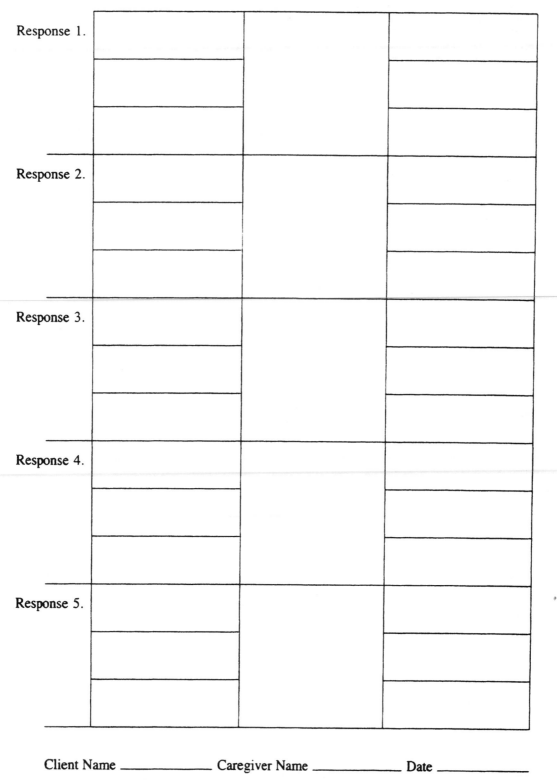

Response 1.

Response 2.

Response 3.

Response 4.

Response 5.

Client Name _____ Caregiver Name _____ Date _____

Level _____ Lesson _____ Therapist _____ Comments _____

_____

Index

DATE DUE

SEP 1 5 1999	